THE
HARVARD MEDICAL
SCHOOL GUIDE TO

A Good Night's
Sleep

Also from Harvard Medical School

The Harvard Medical School Guide to Healthy Eating During Pregnancy, by W. Allan Walker, M.D., with Courtney Humphries

The Harvard Medical School Guide to Achieving Optimal Memory, by Aaron P. Nelson, Ph.D., with Susan Gilbert

The Harvard Medical School Guide to Lowering Your Cholesterol, by Mason W. Freeman, M.D., with Christine Junge

The Harvard Medical School Guide to Healing Your Sinuses, by Ralph B. Metson, M.D., with Steven Mardon

The Harvard Medical School Guide to Overcoming Thyroid Problems, by Jeffrey R. Garber, M.D., with Sandra Sardella White

The Harvard Medical School Guide to Lowering Your Blood Pressure, by Aggie Casey, R.N., M.S., and Herbert Benson, M.D., with Brian O'Neill

Living Through Breast Cancer, by Carolyn M. Kaelin, M.D., M.P.H., with Francesca Coltrera

The Breast Cancer Survivor's Fitness Plan, by Carolyn M. Kaelin, M.D., M.P.H., Francesca Coltrera, Josie Gardiner, and Joy Prouty

Hot Flashes, Hormones, and Your Health, by JoAnne E. Manson, M.D., with Shari S. Bassuk, Sc.D.

Beating Diabetes, by David M. Nathan, M.D., and Linda Delahanty, M.S., RD

Eat, Play, and Be Healthy, by W. Allan Walker, M.D., with Courtney Humphries

The No Sweat Exercise Plan, by Harvey B. Simon, M.D.

THE
HARVARD MEDICAL
SCHOOL GUIDE TO

A Good Night's
Sleep

LAWRENCE J. EPSTEIN, M.D.,
WITH STEVEN MARDON

Mc
Graw

New York Chicago San Francisco Lisbon London Madrid Mexico City
Milan New Delhi San Juan Seoul Singapore Sydney Toronto

Library of Congress Cataloging-in-Publication Data

Epstein, Lawrence (Lawrence L. J.)
    The Harvard Medical School guide to a good night's sleep / by Lawrence J. Epstein
and Steven Mardon.
       p.   cm.
    Includes index.
    ISBN 0-07-146743-2
    1. Sleep disorders—Popular works.   I. Mardon, Steven.   II. Title.

    RC547.E67   2007
    616.8'498—dc22   2006021415

1 2 3 4 5 6 7 8 9 10 11 12 13 14 15 16 17 18 19 20   DOC/DOC   0 9 8 7 6

ISBN-13: 978-0-07-146743-8
ISBN-10:   0-07-146743-2

Interior design by Think Design Group, LLC
Interior artwork on pages 14, 19, and 21 by Harriet Greenfield, on page 132 by Scott Leighton, and on page 136 by Doron Ben-Ami

McGraw-Hill books are available at special quantity discounts to use as premiums and sales promotions, or for use in corporate training programs. For more information, please write to the Director of Special Sales, Professional Publishing, McGraw-Hill, Two Penn Plaza, New York, NY 10121-2298. Or contact your local bookstore.

The information contained in this book is intended to provide helpful and informative material on the subject addressed. It is not intended to serve as a replacement for professional medical advice. Any use of the information in this book is at the reader's discretion. The author, publisher, and the President and Fellows of Harvard College specifically disclaim any and all liability arising directly or indirectly from the use or application of any information contained in this book. A health care professional should be consulted regarding your specific situation.

This book is printed on acid-free paper.

To my parents, Stanley and Rosebel, who made it all possible, and to Dorothy, Collin, and Evan, whose love and support made it doable

Contents

Preface   xiii

Acknowledgments   xv

PART I

Understanding The Need for Sleep

CHAPTER 1   3

Good Sleep: An Essential Element of Health

You Are Not Alone   4

Poor Sleep Is a Serious Problem   5

Dramatic Improvements in Diagnosis and Treatment   7

Setting Realistic Expectations   8

CHAPTER 2   11

The ABCs of Zs: What Happens During Sleep?

Sleep and Brain Waves   11

Sleep Architecture   18

The Sleep/Wake Symphony   19

The Sleep Conductor at Work   24

CHAPTER 3   27

How Much Sleep Do I Need—And What Happens If I Don't Get Enough?

Short, Standard, and Long Sleepers   27

Larks and Owls   30

Types of Sleep Deprivation   32

Sleep as a Part of a Healthy Lifestyle   35

Benefits of Sleep   37

CHAPTER 4   39

Sleep and Age: Why Can't I Sleep Like I Used To?

Childhood   39

Adulthood   42

From Sixty On   45

The Big Picture   46

CHAPTER 5   49

Sleep Myths and Facts

You Need Less Sleep as You Get Older   49

Alcohol Helps You Sleep Better   50

Snoring Is Annoying but Harmless   50

There's Something Wrong If You Don't Remember Your Dreams   50

I Can Get by Fine on Five or Six Hours of Sleep   51

You Can Learn to Get by on Less Sleep   51

Insomniacs Barely Sleep at All   51

Falling Asleep During the Day Is a Sign of Laziness   52

Listening to Self-Help Recordings While You Sleep Can Help You Learn   52

Napping Is a Bad Habit   53

It's Possible to Get Too Much Sleep   53

How I Sleep Doesn't Affect the Rest of My Health   54

CHAPTER 6   55

How to Get a Good Night's Sleep: A Six-Step Plan

Recognize the Importance of Sleep   56

Adopt a Healthy Lifestyle   56

Maintain Good Sleep Habits   58

Create the Optimal Sleep Environment   61

Watch Out for Sleep Saboteurs   62

Seek Help for Persistent Sleep Problems   65

PART II

Sleep Disorders and Their Treatments

CHAPTER 7   69

Signs of a Sleep Problem

I Can't Fall Asleep	70
I Can't Stay Awake	74
I Can't Get Up in the Morning	75
I Do Strange Things in My Sleep	76
I Can't Sleep Because of My Partner	78

CHAPTER 8   79

Insomnia and Its Behavioral Treatments

Defining and Classifying Insomnia	79
Behavioral Treatments for Insomnia	83

CHAPTER 9   95

Medications for Treating Insomnia

What Separates One Sleeping Pill from Another	96
Over-the-Counter Medications	99
Prescription Medications	101
My Perspective on Sleep Medication	110

CHAPTER 10   115

Alternative Insomnia Treatments

Herbal Supplements	116
Synthetic Melatonin	119
Acupuncture	120
Hot Baths	121

CHAPTER 11   123

Sleep-Related Breathing Disorders: Snoring and Sleep Apnea

Simple Snoring	124
Obstructive Sleep Apnea	130
Central Sleep Apnea	140

CHAPTER 12   143

Movement Disorders: Restless Legs and Periodic Limb Movements

Restless Legs Syndrome   143

Periodic Limb Movement Disorder   151

CHAPTER 13   153

Narcolepsy

Causes of Narcolepsy   153

Symptoms of Narcolepsy   155

Diagnosis   159

Treatment   161

Living with Narcolepsy   164

CHAPTER 14   167

Parasomnias: Sleepwalking and Other Unusual Behaviors

Deep Sleep Parasomnias   168

REM Parasomnias   172

Other Parasomnias   176

CHAPTER 15   181

Disturbances of Sleep Timing: DSP and ASP

Symptoms of Delayed and Advanced Sleep Phase Disorders   182

Treatments for DSP and ASP   185

CHAPTER 16   191

Challenging Sleep Situations: Jet Lag, Shift Work, and Drowsy Driving

Jet Lag   191

Shift Work   196

Drowsy Driving   204

CHAPTER 17   209

My Child Doesn't Sleep Well, So I Don't Either

Newborns and Infants   210

Toddlers   217

Preschoolers 219

Young Children 222

Adolescents 225

CHAPTER 18 229

Diagnosis: What to Expect from a Sleep Doctor or Sleep Center

When Should I See a Doctor About My Sleep? 229

Seeing a Sleep Doctor 231

The Sleep Center 236

Getting Your Diagnosis 240

CHAPTER 19 243

Health Conditions and Medications That Disrupt Sleep

Cardiovascular Disease 243

Endocrine Disorders 245

Neurological Disorders 247

Respiratory Disease 250

Mental Illness 251

Other Health Problems 253

Medications That Disturb Sleep and Wakefulness 254

Good Night and Good Luck 257

Additional Resources 259

Index 261

Preface

Why would I write a book on sleep? After all, everyone sleeps, it looks easy, and nothing much seems to happen while you're doing it. That's what I used to think before I started studying sleep. I first came across the intricacies and mysteries of sleep as an undergraduate studying psychobiology at UCLA in the 1970s. I was amazed at how much was actually happening during what most people think of as downtime or wasted hours. Still more fascinating was the emerging idea that time spent asleep was essential to proper functioning. As we gained more knowledge, it became clearer that proper sleep plays a large role in maintaining health, promoting learning, performing at top proficiency, and sustaining emotional well-being.

In some ways, this shouldn't be a mystery. Anything we devote a third of our lives to must be important. Just about every animal we have looked at shows periods of sleep. The sleep of all mammals is very similar to our own, differing only in the amount of time spent asleep. Even birds show a rapid eye movement (REM)/non-REM cycle similar to ours.

Sleep is a complex undertaking, requiring numerous pathways through multiple parts of the brain. Several of these areas seem to function just to direct other regions. Every multistep process in the body is vulnerable to potential problems at any point in that process. It is these problems that cause disease, and the same is true with sleep. Given its complexity, the true mystery is that most of the time everything works correctly.

This brings me back to how I've come to write this book. After my first exposure to studying sleep, I filed my interest away and went on with my education, finishing college and medical school. But I didn't learn about sleep and sleep disorders in medical school. That didn't happen until I was doing my residency in internal medicine and found out about a sleep disorder called sleep apnea. To understand this disorder, I had to learn about sleep again, which rekindled my interest.

At that time, the only way to study sleep disorders was to do so as part of another field. I chose pulmonary and critical care medicine at Cedars-Sinai Medical Center in Los Angeles, where Dr. Philip R. Westbrook had just arrived from the Mayo Clinic to set up a sleep disorders center. Under his tutelage, I learned about the different sleep systems, the various disorders, and the available treatments. I also learned what a big impact poor sleep and sleep deprivation have on people. This was probably the most valuable lesson—sleep is important in maintaining good health and enjoying life.

There continues to be much to learn. My time working at Sleep HealthCenters has given me the opportunity to be part of the Harvard Medical School system and interact with some of the foremost experts in sleep physiology, circadian rhythms, and sleep medicine. I work in a truly exciting place, and I am indebted to all of my colleagues who continue to educate me.

An important part of my job is to educate others, both physicians and patients, about the value of good sleep. I do this by seeing patients in a clinic setting, giving talks, writing papers, and preparing videos and slide sets. It's also as simple as telling people at a party what I do for a living. Invariably the response I get is, "Boy, do I need to talk to you!" I have found that a lot of people need and want to learn how to sleep better.

So when Dr. Anthony Komaroff at Harvard Health Publications invited me to write this book, it was a great opportunity to continue to get the message out. My goal was to create a source the reader could come to for general information as well as specific steps for identifying and solving problems. I hope this book stimulates your interest and also helps you improve your sleep.

Acknowledgments

The timing for this book couldn't be better. Sleep medicine has come into its own with increased scientific and clinical interest in sleep and sleep disorders. There has also been a surge in the general public's interest in sleep and the need for materials to explain new discoveries. This convergence of new science and public interest served as the impetus for writing this book.

The book is based on the work of multiple pioneers in sleep medicine who had the vision to explore areas that others thought was uninteresting and unrewarding. I would like to thank those who sparked my interest in sleep medicine and taught me the lessons that continue to guide my practice and ongoing education, particularly Adrian J. Williams, M.D., and Philip R. Westbrook, M.D.

I would like to acknowledge the contributions of Dorothy J. Cunningham, M.D., Stephen O. Sheldon, D.O., and Cynthia Dorsey, Ph.D., who added valuable advice and editing. I also must thank the American Academy of Sleep Medicine, as well as its executive director, Jerry Barrett, for providing me with several of the figures in this book. Finding the time to work on this project while still maintaining my practice would not have been possible without the support of Paul S. Valentine, CEO, David P. White, M.D., and the staff at Sleep HealthCenters. I would also like to thank my coauthor, Steven Mardon, who contributed mightily, was great to work with, and persevered during the tough parts.

PART I

Understanding
The Need for Sleep

CHAPTER 1

Good Sleep: An Essential Element of Health

Some nights, sleep comes easily, and you cruise through the night with minimal interruption. Waking up after a night of good sleep is wonderful—you feel refreshed, energized, and ready to take on the world. Other nights, sleep comes slowly or not until the early morning hours. Or you may fall asleep, only to awaken throughout the night.

As you probably know from experience, sleepless nights often trigger a series of unwanted events. Merely getting out of bed when the alarm goes off can seem like a Herculean task. You may snap at your spouse over cereal for something trivial. At work, you may lack motivation to do normally enjoyable tasks. Perhaps you doze off while watching the evening news—just before the segment you most wanted to see. A few hours later, it's time to go to bed again, and you're faced with the uncertainty of whether you're in for another night of tossing and turning. How can something so right go so wrong?

In this book, I'll help you find the answer. You'll understand what happens during sleep, what can go wrong, and how you can help yourself get a truly good night's sleep.

Too often we forget that sleep is a basic physiological drive, like hunger or thirst, and necessary for life and proper functioning. Those who don't pay attention to ensuring they get adequate, restful sleep can suffer ill health and enjoy life less. I've treated people with sleep problems for more than fifteen years, and I've found that the overwhelming majority of individuals can get better sleep—if they're willing to make sleep a priority, identify the source of their sleep problem (possibly with a physician's assistance), and then follow through on the recommended treatment.

There is much to look forward to, but before we dive in, I'd like to start by raising a few key points about sleep.

You Are Not Alone

If you don't sleep as well as you'd like to, you have plenty of company. A 2005 survey by the National Sleep Foundation (NSF) found that, during the preceding year, 75 percent of adults had at least one symptom of a sleep problem, such as waking a lot during the night or snoring, and 54 percent experienced at least one symptom of insomnia. Here are some additional statistics:

- An estimated 30 to 40 percent of the U.S. population suffers occasionally from insomnia, with 10 to 15 percent having a chronic problem.
- Forty percent of adults snore; 2 to 4 percent suffer from obstructive sleep apnea (pauses in breathing during sleep); and about 5 to 10 percent have restless legs syndrome (RLS), causing them to experience painful or unpleasant tingling in their legs at night.
- The partner of someone with a sleep disorder often experiences sleep that is just as disrupted as that of the person with the disorder. For instance, researchers at the Mayo Clinic found that treating one person's sleep apnea and snoring allowed his or her spouse to get, on average, an hour

more of sleep each night during the same amount of time in bed.

- Americans average 6.9 hours of sleep a night—less than the 7.5 to 8 hours sleep experts believe most people need to function at their best.
- Each year, Americans spend an estimated $2 billion on sleep medications and make almost two million overnight visits to sleep laboratories.

The number of Americans diagnosed and treated for sleep problems has risen in recent years and is expected to continue to grow in the future. Some of this is due to increased awareness— more patients are going to their doctors with sleep complaints and more doctors now recognize the signs of sleep disorders. But other factors—the increasingly hectic pace of modern life, the rising prevalence of obesity, and the aging of the population— may also be contributing to a genuine increase in the percentage of people with sleep problems.

Poor Sleep Is a Serious Problem

We pay a high price for getting an insufficient amount of sleep, individually and as a society:

- Lack of sleep is directly linked to poor health, with new research suggesting it increases the risk of diabetes, heart disease, and obesity. A study published in the journal *Sleep* in 2004 found that women who averaged less than five hours of sleep per night had a significantly higher death rate than those who slept seven hours.
- Even a few nights of bad sleep can be detrimental. One study found that people who were limited to three straight nights of sleeping five hours or less were more likely to have physical ailments such as headaches, stomach problems, and sore joints. Other studies have shown that curtailing sleep to

four hours a night for several nights results in changes in metabolism that are similar to those that occur in normal aging and that raise levels of hormones linked with overeating and weight gain.

- Sleep debt is cumulative. Studies have shown that performance on tests of alertness and thinking continues to get worse the longer sleep deprivation lasts. In other words, we do not adapt to sleep deprivation.

- The combination of sleep deprivation and driving can have deadly consequences. Nearly one in five drivers admits to having fallen asleep at the wheel, and the National Highway Traffic Safety Administration conservatively estimates that one hundred thousand police-reported crashes are caused by drowsy drivers each year, causing seventy-six thousand injuries and fifteen thousand deaths.

- Sleep deprivation played a role in catastrophes such as the Exxon *Valdez* oil spill off the coast of Alaska, the space shuttle *Challenger* disaster, and the nuclear accident at Three Mile Island.

- Sleep deprivation and sleep disorders are estimated to cost Americans over $100 billion annually in lost productivity, medical expenses, sick leave, and property and environmental damage.

Even when sleep deprivation does not cause illness or accidents, it can affect your quality of life. Sleep problems affect virtually every aspect of day-to-day living, such as your mood, mental alertness, work performance, and energy level. According to the 2005 NSF survey, almost three in ten working adults say they have missed work or made errors at work because of sleep-related issues in the past three months. And nearly one-fourth of partnered adults say they have sex less often or have lost interest in sex because they are too sleepy.

Unfortunately, despite some recent progress, fewer than 3 percent of Americans with sleep problems get treatment because both patients and their primary care doctors often do not consider sleep an important health issue. This is partly due to lack of training for physicians and partly because many people accept poor sleep as inevitable.

A survey of American medical schools in 1990 showed that 37 percent did not offer any training in sleep medicine. As recently as 1998, the average amount of sleep education averaged a little more than two hours during the four years of medical school. As a result, doctors frequently fail to ask patients about their sleep.

On the patient side, people with sleep problems often do not report them to their physicians. They believe poor sleep is not a medical problem and incorrectly assume it is normal to feel tired throughout the day or have difficulty getting to sleep at night.

The good news is that this situation is starting to change. Medical training institutions are adding sleep medicine training programs, sleep medicine is now recognized as an official medical subspecialty, and physicians can demonstrate their proficiency by taking board-certification examinations. Between 1993 and 2003, the number of physicians certified in sleep medicine increased more than six-fold to nearly two thousand.

Health and regulatory officials, as well as the general public, are also starting to wake up to the importance of sleep. For example, some school districts, urged on by frustrated parents, have changed starting times for classes to make them more amenable to adolescents' natural sleep patterns. In New Jersey, drowsy driving is now treated as a criminal offense similar to driving while intoxicated; other states are considering following suit.

Dramatic Improvements in Diagnosis and Treatment

Much has happened in recent decades to make it easier to recognize and treat sleep problems.

Diagnosis

Sleep disorders are now more easily diagnosed, thanks to a better understanding of patient needs and improvements in technology.

Overnight sleep centers are now designed to resemble hotels rather than hospitals, making patients feel more comfortable. The monitoring equipment is more sensitive than in the past, making for more accurate diagnoses. And computerization and miniaturization have led to the development of equipment so small and light that testing can sometimes be done at home rather than at a sleep center.

Medication

We have a larger and more effective arsenal to treat sleep problems today than we did even five years ago. Today's drugs for insomnia are safer and less likely to cause morning grogginess or lead to dependence. There are now several classes of potent medications useful in treating RLS, and we are on the verge of finding medical treatments for narcolepsy that may cure the disorder rather than just treat its symptoms.

Hi-Tech Treatments

The devices used to treat sleep disorders are more effective now because of better materials and improved designs. For example, positive airway pressure (PAP), the primary treatment for sleep apnea, can now be tailored to a particular patient's facial shape, and the new equipment is smaller, lighter, and designed to make travel easier. Oral appliances for snoring have also improved. Surgery, a last resort for sleep apnea and snoring, has advanced with the use of lasers, radio frequency waves, and plastic stents. Many procedures can now be done in an office setting with only local anesthesia. Light, focused on the back of the eye, can be used to reset the internal clock and treat circadian rhythm disorders such as jet lag. As sleep disorders receive more attention, treatments will continue to advance, improving both comfort and success.

Setting Realistic Expectations

As we start this journey, what should you expect? Will you be able to sleep as well today as you did as a child? Will you learn to fall asleep in two minutes every night without fail? Probably not. But you can look forward to improving the quality and quantity of the sleep you get each night and, as a result, how you feel during the day.

To start out, you'll learn about normal sleep, which will allow you to recognize if what you are experiencing is a genuine problem or not. Perhaps it's not—as you'll see, it's not abnormal to have trouble falling or staying asleep on occasion, especially as you age.

But if you do have a problem, you'll learn to identify it and then find the appropriate treatment strategy or remedy. If your trouble stems from failing to make enough time for sleep or from flaws in your sleep environment, then adjusting your routine and correcting the fault may be the solution. If you find you have a sleep disorder, you'll need to get appropriate treatment.

Regardless of the problem's source, addressing it should improve your sleep and your daytime energy and alertness. You'll be less likely to doze off unexpectedly at the movies or while watching TV, and you should see quality of life improvements such as reduced sick days, higher energy, and better mental health. It's not uncommon for a patient I've treated to tell me he or she feels like a whole new person.

Before you can identify and address what's causing your difficulties, you need an understanding of the ABCs of sleep. So in Part I of this book, we'll explore exactly what happens physiologically when you sleep and the different factors that can cause sleep problems. You'll need that fundamental knowledge as we move on to Part II, which covers the different sleep disorders and range of available treatments.

CHAPTER 2

The ABCs of Zs: What Happens During Sleep?

Given how much time we spend sleeping, it's remarkable how little many of us know about what actually happens to our brains and bodies during sleep. While there's no need for you to be an expert on sleep physiology to address your own sleep difficulties, the more you understand about the need for sleep and the mechanics of good sleep, the better able you'll be to prevent sleep problems from developing, fix problems that do occur, and know when to seek help to treat a sleep disorder.

It's time for Sleep 101. But don't worry, there won't be a quiz at the end of the chapter.

Sleep and Brain Waves

For many centuries, scientists scrutinized minute aspects of human activity but showed little interest in the time that people spent sleeping. Sleep seemed inaccessible to medical probing and was perceived as a passive state in which both the body and the brain were quiet and unresponsive—a subject best suited to poets and dream interpreters who could conjure meaning out of the void.

That changed in the 1930s, when scientists discovered that chemical reactions in the brain produced waves of electrical current that could be detected on the surface of the body. The next step was to place sensitive electrodes on the scalp to capture a recording of electrical activity. Measured in cycles per second, this recording is called an electroencephalogram (EEG). Originally recorded on paper charts, today's tracings from an EEG go directly into a computer.

The size and frequency of brain waves varies depending on where in the brain the waves originate, how alert the person is, and how urgent the message being transmitted is. These different states produce brain waves of varying speed (fast and slow) and size (large and small). As a result, the picture of brain activity displayed on an EEG changes constantly from fast, small waves when a person is active or engaged in specific mental activities to large, slow waves when he or she is resting or in deep sleep.

To understand the recording of brain waves, imagine yourself standing on the edge of a pond. You throw in a small stone, which causes a ripple of waves spreading out from the center to all sides of the pond. The electrical activity of the different brain centers acts like the stone, causing waves to spread throughout the brain.

The pattern of waves in the pond changes as you toss in more stones. With a single stone, you generate large, regular waves. If you throw a handful of stones, the waves they generate interfere with each other, causing the pattern to be more jumbled. Similarly, the EEG pattern depends on what's happening in the brain at the time of observation. When multiple activity centers are processing information and firing, the brain waves interfere with each other, and the resulting waves are small, irregular, and chaotic looking. The more active the brain, the more small, fast, irregular waves are seen. The EEG of a less active brain shows a larger, slower, and more regular wave pattern.

After a few years of brain wave study, it became clear that sleep was a highly complex and dynamic activity. The brain was not passively and uniformly shutting down during sleep but rather passing through several different patterns of activity in an orderly fashion. Scientists now describe several discrete stages of sleep based on different combinations of brain wave patterns, eye movements, and muscle tone. Researchers are continually learning more about the unique role certain stages of sleep play in maintaining health, growth, and daytime functioning.

Scientists divide sleep into two major types:

* Non-REM, or quiet, sleep
* Rapid eye movement (REM), or dreaming, sleep

Surprisingly, they are as different from one another as sleeping is from waking.

Quiet Sleep

Sleep specialists have called non-REM sleep "an idling brain in a movable body." During this phase, thinking and most physiological activities slow down, but movement can still occur, and a person often shifts position while sinking into progressively deeper stages of sleep.

To an extent, the convention of describing people "descending" or "dropping" into sleep actually parallels changes in brain wave patterns at the onset of non-REM sleep. When you are awake, billions of brain cells receive and analyze sensory information, coordinate behavior, and maintain bodily functions by sending electrical impulses to one another, which can be recorded as brain waves. Similar to our example of a handful of stones thrown into a pond, the multitude of different waves generated when we're fully awake interfere with each other, cancel each other out, and result in the EEG recording an irregular scribble of electrical activity, as shown in Figure 2.1.

Alpha Sleep. Once your eyes are closed and your nerve cells no longer receive visual input, brain waves settle into a steady and rhythmic pattern of about eight to twelve cycles per second. This

FIGURE 2.1 Brain Wave Patterns During Sleep

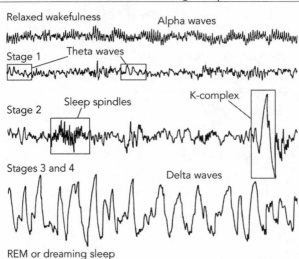

Brain waves, recorded on an electroencephalogram, are used to identify the stages of sleep. Alpha waves emerge during relaxed wakefulness with the eyes closed. The change to Stage 1 sleep is marked by loss of alpha waves and the appearance of theta waves. The hallmarks of Stage 2 sleep are brief bursts of activity, called sleep spindles, and K-complex waves. Deep sleep (Stages 3 and 4) is represented by large, slow delta waves.

is the alpha wave pattern, characteristic of calm, relaxed wakefulness. Unless something disturbs the process, you will soon proceed smoothly through the four stages of non–REM sleep.

Stage 1. In making the transition from wakefulness into light sleep, you spend about five minutes in Stage 1 sleep. On the EEG, the predominant brain waves slow to four to seven cycles per second, a pattern called theta waves. Body temperature begins to drop, muscles become relaxed, and eyes often move slowly from side to side. People in Stage 1 sleep lose awareness of their surroundings, but they are easily jarred into wakefulness. However, not everyone experiences Stage 1 sleep in the same way; if awakened, one person might recall being only drowsy, while another might describe having been asleep.

Stage 2. This is the first stage of established sleep. The first time it occurs it lasts ten to twenty-five minutes before you progress to another stage of sleep. Your eyes are usually still, and your heart rate and breathing are slower than when you're awake. Your brain's electrical activity is irregular. Intermediate-size brain waves intermingle with brief bursts of fast activity called sleep spindles, when brain waves speed up for roughly half a second or longer. About every two minutes, EEG tracings show a pattern called a K-complex, which scientists think represents a sort of built-in vigilance system that keeps you poised to be awakened if necessary. K-complexes can be provoked by certain sounds or other external or internal stimuli. Whisper someone's name during Stage 2 sleep, and a K-complex will appear on the EEG. Stage 2 sleep is commonly seen in the transition between other sleep stages; overall, about half the night is usually spent in Stage 2 sleep.

Stages 3 and 4, or Deep Sleep. As you travel into deeper sleep, fewer and fewer of the brain's processing centers stay active and the firing of the remaining active brain cells becomes more coordinated. From our pond example, this would be like when your supply of stones starts to run out and you throw fewer at a time and less frequently, finally throwing only one at a time to keep from running out. The resulting waves become bigger and more distinct. Eventually, large slow brain waves called delta waves become the major feature on the EEG.

Together, Stages 3 and 4 are known as deep sleep, or slow-wave sleep. Stage 4 sleep occurs when at least half of the brain waves are delta waves. During deep sleep, your breathing slows and becomes more regular. Your blood pressure and pulse fall to about 20 to 30 percent below their waking rates. Your brain becomes less responsive to external stimuli, making it difficult to awaken.

Deep sleep seems to be a time for your body to renew and repair itself. Less blood flow is directed toward your brain, which cools measurably. At the beginning of this stage, the pituitary gland releases a pulse of growth hormone that stimulates tissue

Why Do We Dream?

You've probably wondered whether your dreams serve any purpose. What does it mean when you dream of arriving at your senior prom in overalls or being chased through the streets of Paris by a giant turtle?

Researchers who have studied dreaming fall into two camps: those who believe that dreams are important, and those who believe they're not. Members of the first camp can trace their ideas to Sigmund Freud, who in 1900 proposed that dreams are meaningful representations of the unconscious mind in which we reveal our hidden conflicts, desires, and fears, albeit in disguised form. Post-Freudian theorists and psychoanalytic thinkers subsequently elaborated on and refined his ideas, focusing on how dreams help the organization of thought and the consolidation and reinforcement of long-term memory.

Other researchers, taking a physiological approach, are skeptical. Pointing to studies from the 1970s showing that dreams occur upon activation of neurotransmitter chemicals in a portion of the brain, they argue that dreams are little more than the mind's

growth and muscle repair. Researchers have also detected increased blood levels of substances such as interleukin that activate your immune system, raising the possibility that deep sleep helps the body defend itself against infection.

Normally, young adults spend about 20 percent of their sleep time in up to half-hour stretches of slow-wave sleep, but slow-wave sleep declines sharply in most people over age sixty-five. When a sleep-deprived person finally gets some sleep, he or she passes quickly through the lighter sleep stages into the deeper stages and spends a greater proportion there, suggesting that slow-wave sleep is the restorative portion of sleep you need to feel refreshed.

attempt to make meaning out of the random chemical signals sent up from the brain stem. They also point out that we only remember a minute percentage of our dreams; if they were significant, surely we'd remember more.

Current research on the function of dreams combines features of both the psychological and neurochemical approaches. One study, for example, observed that patients who sustained injuries and lesions in the brain's frontal lobe (not the brain stem) no longer dreamed. This suggests that parts of the brain other than the brain stem—specifically those areas in the front of the brain that are connected to urges, impulses, and appetites—may be involved in dream production, and it has prompted a reexamination of the Freudian notion that dreams may represent a window to a person's emotions.

Dreaming is clearly involved in memory and learning so it performs a useful and necessary function. Research in coming decades should offer important insights on why we dream and what role our dreams can play in maintaining mental health.

Dreaming Sleep

Dreaming occurs during REM sleep, which has been described as an "active brain in a paralyzed body." Your brain races as your eyes dart back and forth rapidly behind closed lids. Your body temperature rises. Unless you have circulatory or other physical problems, the penis or clitoris becomes erect. Your blood pressure increases, and your heart rate and breathing speed up to daytime levels. The sympathetic nervous system, which creates the fight-or-flight response, is twice as active as when you're awake. Despite all this activity, your body hardly moves except for intermittent twitches, because muscles not needed for breathing or eye movement are temporarily paralyzed.

We don't know whether dreams have deep meaning. But we do know that just as deep sleep restores your body, dreaming sleep restores your mind, perhaps in part by helping clear out irrelevant information. Studies show, for example, that REM sleep facilitates learning and memory. People tested to measure how well they have learned a new task improve their scores after a night's sleep. If repeatedly roused from REM sleep, however, the improvements are lost. On the other hand, if they are awakened an equal number of times from slow-wave sleep, the improvements in the scores are unaffected. Such findings may help explain why students who stay up all night cramming for an examination generally retain less information than classmates who get some sleep.

Three to five times a night, or about every ninety minutes, a sleeper enters REM sleep. The first such episode usually lasts for only a few minutes, but REM time increases progressively over the course of the night. The final period of REM sleep may last half an hour. Altogether, REM sleep makes up about 25 percent of total sleep in young adults. If someone who has been deprived of REM sleep is left undisturbed for a night, he or she enters this stage earlier and spends a higher proportion of sleep time in it—a phenomenon called REM rebound.

Sleep Architecture

During the night, a normal sleeper moves between different sleep stages in a fairly predictable pattern, alternating between REM and non-REM sleep. When these stages are charted on a diagram, called a hypnogram, the different levels resemble a drawing of a city skyline, as shown in Figure 2.2. Sleep experts call this pattern sleep architecture.

In a young adult, normal sleep architecture usually consists of four or five alternating non-REM and REM periods. Most deep sleep occurs in the first half of the night; as the night progresses, periods of REM sleep get longer and alternate with Stage 2 sleep. Later in life, the sleep skyline will change, with less deep sleep,

FIGURE 2.2 Sleep Architecture

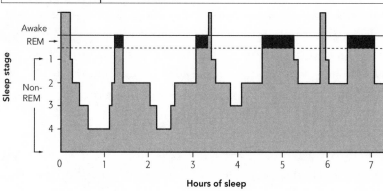

The hypnogram is a chart of sleep stages over the course of the night and resembles a drawing of a city skyline. This pattern is known as sleep architecture. This hypogram shows a typical night's sleep.

more Stage 1 sleep, and more awakenings. We'll talk more about how sleep changes as you age in the next chapter.

The Sleep/Wake Symphony

When it's working well, the sleep process seems like a finely tuned orchestra, with various sections of the brain sounding off at just the right time. How is this orchestra conducted? What keeps the various parts in tune and in synch? To answer these questions, we need to examine the brain structures and external factors that produce this symphony of alternating states of sleep and wakefulness in the first place.

Several physiological processes are involved in the sleep/wake symphony, in particular circadian rhythms and the sleep-inducing drive called homeostasis.

Circadian Rhythms and Your Internal Clock

A pacemaker-like mechanism in the brain regulates the daily routine of sleeping and waking. This internal clock—also known as the biological clock—gradually becomes established during the first months of life. It controls the ups and downs of physiological patterns, including body temperature, blood pressure, the release of hormones (such as melatonin and cortisol), digestive-juice secretion, urine production, and the timing of sleep and wakefulness. Each of these patterns and dozens more have a daily rhythm. Accordingly, we call them circadian rhythms, from the Latin phrase meaning "about a day."

The circadian rhythm of sleep and wakefulness—the sleep/wake rhythm, for short—makes your desire for sleep strongest between midnight and dawn, and also strong in midafternoon. This is called a bimodal, or two-peaked, pattern, as shown in Figure 2.3. The highest peak of sleepiness occurs in the early morning hours. A second small peak occurs twelve hours later, in the middle of the afternoon. This is the physiological basis for the traditional siesta, or afternoon nap. In one study, researchers instructed a group of people to try to stay awake for twenty-four hours. Not surprisingly, many slipped into naps despite their best efforts not to. When the investigators plotted the times the unplanned naps occurred, they found peaks between 2 A.M. and 4 A.M. and between 2 P.M. and 3 P.M.

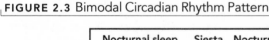

FIGURE 2.3 Bimodal Circadian Rhythm Pattern

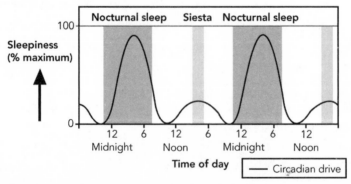

The circadian rhythm of sleep and wakefulness makes a person's desire for sleep strongest between midnight and dawn, with a second smaller peak in the middle of the afternoon. Source: Adapted from M. M. Mitler et al., "Methods of Testing for Sleepiness," *Behavioral Medicine* 21, 1996: 171–83.

Most Americans sleep only during the night, as dictated by their sleep/wake rhythm, although many nap in the afternoon on the weekends. In societies where taking a siesta is the norm, people can respond to their bodies' daily dips in alertness with a one- to two-hour afternoon nap during the workday and a correspondingly shorter sleep at night.

In the 1970s, the location of the internal clock was found to be the suprachiasmatic nucleus (SCN). This cluster of cells is part of the hypothalamus, the brain center that regulates appetite and other biological states. When this tiny area was damaged in laboratory rodents, the sleep/wake rhythm disappeared and they no longer slept on a normal schedule. Figure 2.4 shows the location of the SCN within the hypothalamus, just beneath the nerve tracts that take information from the eyes to the visual centers of

FIGURE 2.4 Sleep/Wake Control Center

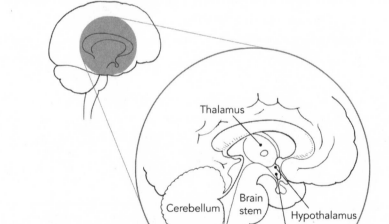

The pacemaker-like mechanism in your brain that regulates the circadian rhythm of sleep and wakefulness is located in the suprachiasmatic nucleus. This cluster of cells is part of the hypothalamus, the brain center that regulates appetite, body temperature, and other biological states.

the brain. The retina of the eye connects to the SCN, which helps explain the influence of light on circadian rhythms.

Zeitgebers

Although largely self-regulating, the clock responds to several types of external clues to keep it set at twenty-four hours. Scientists call these cues zeitgebers, a German word meaning "time givers." Key zeitgebers include light, time cues, and melatonin.

Light. Light striking your eyes is the most influential zeitgeber. Because of the connections between the eye and the SCN, light can directly affect the sleep/wake rhythm. When researchers exposed volunteers at a sleep lab to light at intervals that were at odds with the outside world, the participants unconsciously reset their biological clocks to match the new light input. Up to 90 percent of blind people have circadian rhythm disturbances and sleep problems, demonstrating the importance of light to sleep/wake patterns. Researchers have learned that delivering pulses of light at specific times during the circadian cycle can cause the rhythm to shift in predictable ways, which is important in treating circadian rhythm disorders.

Time Cues. As a person reads clocks, follows work and transportation schedules, and obeys social demands to remain alert for certain tasks and events, there is continual pressure to stay on schedule. These clues can help the circadian clock adhere to a twenty-four-hour schedule.

Melatonin. Cells in the SCN contain receptors for melatonin, a hormone produced in a predictable daily rhythm by the pineal gland, which is located between the two hemispheres of the brain. In the absence of light, melatonin levels begin climbing in the late evening and ebb after dawn. The production of melatonin can be suppressed, even in the middle of the night, by exposure to light. Scientists believe melatonin's daily light-sensitive cycle helps keep the sleep/wake cycle on track. Large doses of the hormone can induce drowsiness in some people, and melatonin has been shown to help reset the circadian clock, making it useful for adapting to jet lag. We'll cover this in greater detail in Chapter 16.

The Drive for Sleep

Your body has a built-in tendency to maintain internal equilibrium by adjusting its physiological processes—a critical concept known as homeostasis. Homeostasis influences many body functions; for example, if you haven't had anything to drink for a while or sweat while exercising, you get thirsty. In response, you take a drink, replacing the lost fluid, and then you're no longer thirsty. The homeostatic drive also influences the timing of sleep. It has two aspects: elapsed time since last sleep and cumulative sleep debt.

Elapsed Time Since Last Sleep. As you know from experience, the longer you're awake, the more tired you generally feel. A person who typically sleeps from 11 P.M. to 7 A.M. without napping goes sixteen hours between sleep sessions. So as consecutive hours of sleeplessness go beyond this point, the drive for sleep steadily increases. Figure 2.5 shows the homeostatic drive increasing as hours awake accumulate and then decreasing during sleep.

FIGURE 2.5 Homeostatic Sleep Drive

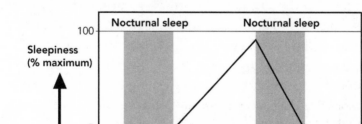

The homeostatic sleep drive increases with consecutive hours of sleeplessness. The straight line represents this drive; note that sleep onset occurs at its peak and then decreases during sleep.

23

Cumulative Sleep Debt. Your body needs a certain amount of sleep to function at its best. For simplicity's sake, let's say it's eight hours. When you fail to get eight hours of sleep, you start to accumulate a sleep debt—somewhat similar to what occurs in your bank account when you regularly withdraw more money than you deposit. If you sleep five hours on Monday, six hours on Tuesday, and seven on Wednesday, then you've built up a sleep debt of six hours $(3 + 2 + 1 = 6)$. The greater your sleep debt over a few days, the stronger the drive for sleep. Your increasing sleepiness is your body's natural attempt to force you to get your eight hours of sleep.

The Sleep Conductor at Work

Whether or not you fall asleep at any given point in time is determined by the interaction of the two aspects of the homeostatic drive, plus what might be called your circadian drive—in other words, the effect of the circadian rhythm of sleep and wakefulness. At times, the circadian and homeostatic drives work together to promote sleep or alertness, as illustrated in Figure 2.6a; at other times, these forces are in opposition, leading to difficulty falling asleep in bed or trouble staying alert during the day, as shown in Figure 2.6b. Let's look at some examples of the rhythms working together.

Say you're at the tail end of a busy week during which you've had no choice but to get up at 6 A.M. and go to bed at midnight. At 12 A.M. on Friday, you've been awake eighteen hours, you've built up a medium-size sleep debt, and it's an ideal time to sleep in terms of the sleep/wake rhythm. Barring unusual circumstances (a sleep disorder, a blaring car alarm, and so on), it shouldn't take you long to fall asleep.

Similarly, at 8:30 P.M. on a weeknight when you've been sleeping well for several days, you should have no problem staying awake, since your circadian and homeostatic drives are both primed for alertness. In fact, conditions are ideal for a superior performance—perhaps you'll jog a mile more than usual, breeze

FIGURE 2.6 Sleep Drives

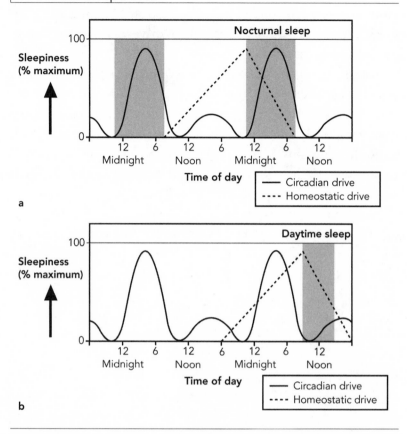

a. The circadian and homeostatic sleep drives are in sync and both peak during the nocturnal sleep period, promoting falling asleep and staying asleep. b. Out-of-sync circadian and homeostatic sleep drives: The circadian drive peaks at night and is lowest in the morning. The homeostatic drive peaks in the morning, promoting daytime sleep, but the opposing circadian drive promotes wakefulness so the resulting daytime sleep is short and often fragmented. This situation occurs commonly with nightshift workers.

through a hundred pages of a novel, or humble your spouse at Scrabble.

Then there are the times when circadian and homeostatic factors are at odds. For example, imagine that you stay up all night after getting up at your usual time. When the sun comes out the following morning, you've been awake more than twenty-four hours, which pushes you toward sleep. But as anyone who's ever worked a night shift knows, circadian rhythms are in wake-up mode at 7 A.M., so you're liable to have trouble falling asleep. In this situation, it's hard to predict which drive will win—it's a battle that can go either way.

Good sleep is best obtained by varying your routine as little as possible. In other words, the best thing you can do to satisfy the drive for sleep is to get enough sleep and to get it during the same time frame each day. The more you defy your body—by staying up for long periods of time, building up a sleep debt, and trying to sleep against the natural drive of the sleep/wake rhythm—the harder it will be to stay awake and fall asleep when you want to.

In the next chapter, we'll tackle the eternal question, "How much sleep do I need?" Then we'll look at the consequences of failing to reach that goal and the benefits of attaining it.

How Much Sleep Do I Need—And What Happens If I Don't Get Enough?

"How much sleep do I need?" is one of the most common questions sleep specialists hear. Often there is a subtle subtext: *Look, Doc, I'm really busy—expanding my company/getting a graduate degree/building an extension on my house/raising three kids—and I can't afford to sleep away one-third of my life. Can't I really get by on four or five hours a night?*

The short answer is: No, you probably can't. But let's explore the question in a little more depth.

Short, Standard, and Long Sleepers

Like many individual traits, such as height, intelligence, and shoe size, the need for sleep among the general population follows a simple bell curve, as shown in Figure 3.1. A few people need a little (four to six hours), a few people need a lot (nine or ten hours), and most are in the middle (seven or eight hours). Most sleep specialists believe the overwhelming majority of people need at least

FIGURE 3.1 Sleep Need in the General Population

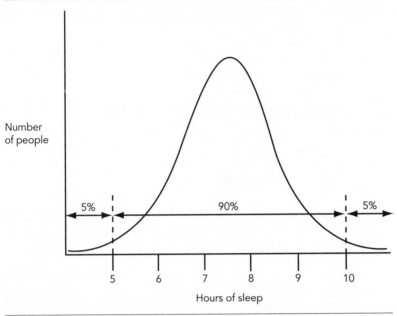

Sleep need among the general population follows a simple bell curve. About 5 percent of people need a little (less than five hours), approximately another 5 percent need a lot (more than ten hours), and the majority need something in between (seven or eight hours).

seven and a half hours of sleep to function at their best. That's a good goal for the average person.

Of course, you want to know your requirements, not those of the average Joe. The best way to calculate your sleep need is to listen to your body. In your experience, how much sleep does it take for you to feel fully rested? By this, I mean you

* find it easy to get out of bed;
* are not sleepy during the daytime;
* don't have problems concentrating; and
* are generally in a good mood.

Conversely, take a minute to think about how much sleep is *not* enough for you. The key here is daytime drowsiness. On days when you feel sleepy during the day, how much sleep did you typically get the night before? Along with feeling drowsy in the daytime, you're probably sleep deprived if you

- struggle to get out of bed;
- are frequently irritable;
- have difficulty concentrating; or
- nod off or come close to nodding off after lunch or dinner, at the movies, watching television, or while driving.

From your experience of being both well rested and sleep deprived, you should be able to get an estimate of how much sleep you truly need. But if you're having trouble coming up with a concrete figure—perhaps because your sleep length is always changing to catch up on lost sleep—it may be easier to make this calculation during a leisurely vacation, when you can set your own hours. Midway through a weeklong break—after repaying some of your sleep debt—you should settle into a routine that meets your body's genuine need. Again, for most people it will be seven and a half to eight hours a day.

Of course, it's possible you'll find you're at one of the extremes. There are some people who genuinely function perfectly well on six hours of sleep a night, and a lucky few who only need five. However, these people—called short sleepers—represent a small percentage of the population. While it's not uncommon to read profiles of well-known businesspeople, historical figures, and celebrities who claim to only sleep four hours a night, often these assertions are unverified and would prove untrue on close inspection. It's likely that many of those who say they don't need much shut-eye compensate for their short sleep with supplemental daytime naps.

Similarly, you might also exist on the opposite end of the spectrum. Some people—"long sleepers"—genuinely need nine or ten hours of sleep a night to function well. Sleeping this much also can be a sign that something's wrong—for example, people with sleep apnea often sleep a lot, and people who are depressed stay in

Sleep in Humans Versus Animals

Compared to other mammals, humans' tendency to sleep seven or eight hours a day falls about in the middle. Here's a listing of the sleep needs of some common animals.

Horse: 3 hours
Cow: 4 hours
Elephant: 4 hours
Giraffe: 4.5 hours
Rabbit: 8 hours
Guinea pig: 9.5 hours
Baboon: 9.5 hours
Dolphin: 10 hours
Dog: 10 hours
Cat: 12.5 hours
Hamster: 14 hours
Sloth: 14.4 hours
Bat: 19 hours

And yes, it's true that horses sleep standing up. However, they can also sleep while lying down.

bed for long periods of time. But sleeping nine or ten hours a night is not in itself a sign of ill health or laziness. (In fact, among many creatures, it's perfectly normal.)

Larks and Owls

Along with sleep length, another aspect of sleep that follows a bell curve is when you feel most comfortable going to bed and waking up. Where these times fall is not a reflection on your character. Instead, it's a nonjudgmental product of your circadian rhythm of sleep and wakefulness. There are three general profiles: standard sleepers, larks, and owls.

- **Standard sleepers.** The sleep/wake rhythm pushes most people to sleep from about 10:30 or 11:30 P.M. to 6:30 or 7:30 A.M.
- **Larks.** A small percentage of people have an inborn tendency to go to bed early and wake up early. Larks feel most comfortable going to bed between 9 and 10 P.M. and waking up between 5 and 6 A.M. These are the people who are most comfortable following Benjamin Franklin's advice about early to bed and early to rise.
- **Owls.** At the other end of the spectrum are the people with a natural desire to go to bed late and sleep late. Owls' late-night tendency makes it easy for them to stay up long past midnight and sleep until the late morning.

As with sleep length, you can most easily determine where you fit in by determining your sleep pattern during a vacation, after you've caught up on any lost sleep.

It's also possible to come up with a precise, scientific classification if you have a thermometer capable of making a round-the-clock record of internal body temperature. The circadian rhythm of body temperature is an effective marker for the sleep/wake cycle and can help you determine if you tend to be a lark or an owl. As you learned in elementary school, body temperature averages 98.6 degrees Fahrenheit. It also fluctuates about one-half of one degree in each direction at various times of the day.

For a person with a standard profile, the absolute low point during the twenty-four-hour period typically comes around 5:30 A.M. By contrast, a lark's temperature minimum occurs around 4:30 A.M., while an owl's strikes shortly before 7 A.M.

One final fact: As we age, we have a tendency to go to sleep earlier and wake up earlier, typically by about an hour. So someone who was an owl as a young man may adopt a standard pattern as a senior citizen, and someone with a standard profile may become a lark. This trend can cause social problems for lifelong larks, since they may find themselves waking up in the predawn hours in their later years.

Types of Sleep Deprivation

The answer to the question, "What happens when I don't get enough sleep?" is more complicated than it might seem. That's because there are actually several different types of sleep deprivation, depending on the duration and severity. We'll broadly break it into complete and partial sleep deprivation.

Complete Sleep Deprivation

Normally, you go about sixteen or seventeen hours between sleep sessions. Complete sleep deprivation is what happens as the hours go beyond this point. The immediate result is you feel tired, and then you feel exhausted. By 2 or 3 A.M., many people have a hard time keeping their eyes open. What's less well known are the effects on your body and its ability to function. Simple tasks that you would have no trouble doing suddenly start to become difficult. In fact, in the past decade, a number of studies on hand-eye coordination and reaction time have shown that such sleep deprivation has a similar effect on human performance to being intoxicated.

In one such study, volunteers were deprived of sleep for twenty-eight hours, beginning at 8 A.M., and then tested on a driving simulator. At a different time, volunteers' driving ability was tested after drinking 10 to 15 grams of alcohol at thirty-minute intervals until their blood alcohol content (BAC) level reached .10. The study concluded that twenty-four hours of wakefulness had the same deleterious effect on driving ability as a BAC of .10—enough to be charged with driving while intoxicated in most states. In addition to poor hand-eye coordination, sleep deprivation also leaves you prone to two potentially dangerous phenomena: microsleeps and automatic behavior.

What happens when complete sleep deprivation is extended for long periods of time? Not surprisingly, things go downhill. Studies have found that when people go two or three days without sleep they have difficulty completing tasks demanding a high attention level and often experience mood swings, depression, and increased feelings of tension.

Microsleeps and Automatic Behavior

Two potentially dangerous phenomena can occur among sleep-deprived people: microsleeps and automatic behavior. Microsleeps are brief episodes of sleep that occur in the midst of ongoing wakeful activity. They typically last a few seconds but can go on for ten or fifteen seconds. Brain wave monitoring by EEG of someone experiencing microsleeps shows brief periods of Stage 1 sleep intruding into wakefulness. During this time, the brain does not attend to sensory input, and you don't respond to things happening in the world around you. The experience people often refer to as nodding off can be the result of a microsleep.

Automatic behavior refers to a period of several minutes or more during which a person is awake and performing routine duties but not attending to their surroundings or responding to changes in the environment. Examples of automatic behavior include a driver who keeps his car on the road but misses his intended exit or a train engineer who can continue pressing a lever at regular intervals but doesn't notice an obstruction on the track.

Microsleeps and automatic behavior play a role in thousands of tragic transportation accidents each year, since a second or two of inattention can be fatal when you're traveling at high speed in a heavy vehicle.

Performance is also highly influenced by fluctuations in circadian rhythms. For example, sleep-deprived people may still function fairly well during the morning and evening. But during the peaks of sleepiness in the afternoon and overnight hours, people often cannot stay awake and may fall asleep while standing; sitting; or even engaging in activities such as talking on the telephone, working on the computer, or eating. A small percentage experience paranoia and hallucinations.

Total sleep deprivation can be dangerous and even fatal. Studies done in the nineteenth century found that puppies deprived of sleep died after seven to ten days, and research conducted in the 1980s found that rats die after two weeks without sleep.

Partial Sleep Deprivation

Partial sleep deprivation is the type that occurs when you get some sleep, but not 100 percent of what you need—what we commonly think of as building up a sleep debt. An example would be when a person who needs seven and a half hours of sleep a night hits a short stretch in which he or she only gets four to six hours.

After a single night of short sleep, most people function at or near their normal level. They may not feel great, but they can usually get through the day without others noticing that anything is amiss.

Problems are more likely to become apparent after two or more nights of short sleep. The most obvious signs are increased irritability and sleepiness. Work performance begins to suffer, particularly on complicated tasks, and people are more likely to complain of headaches, stomach problems, and sore joints. In addition, people are at substantially higher risk of falling asleep on the job and while driving home.

Long-term partial sleep deprivation is what occurs when someone obtains less than the optimal amount of sleep for months or years on end—a common scenario for insomniacs and people with sleep disorders, as well as healthy people who cannot resist taking advantage of the round-the-clock commerce, communication, and entertainment opportunities our 24/7 society now offers. Several studies have associated long-term sleep deficits with significant health problems and shorter life spans:

- A 1979 study of almost a million people over age thirty found that men who reported usually sleeping less than four hours a day were nearly three times as likely to die within six years as men who said they averaged seven or eight hours of sleep.

- A 1983 study at the San Diego Naval School of Health Sciences found that on all performance measures, subjects who slept five to seven hours a day fared worse than those who slept more than seven hours. As a group, poor sleepers received fewer promotions during their careers, stayed at lower pay grades, were less frequently recommended for reenlistment, had a higher attrition rate, and were more likely to be hospitalized during their tour of duty.
- A 2004 study found that women who averaged five hours of sleep a night were 39 percent more likely to develop heart disease than women who got eight hours.
- A different 2004 study found that men limited to four hours of sleep for two consecutive nights experienced hormonal changes—specifically, decreases in the hormone leptin and increases in the peptide ghrelin—that made them feel hungry and crave carbohydrate-rich foods such as cakes, candy, ice cream, and pasta. Researchers feel that constant sleep debt is associated with obesity.

Sleep as Part of a Healthy Lifestyle

As you can see, the consequences of sleep deprivation are serious and potentially even life-threatening, in both the short term (increased accident risk) and the long term (increased disease risk). For this reason, it's vital that you think of getting enough sleep as an essential element of maintaining good health—as important as getting regular exercise, eating a healthy diet, and practicing good dental hygiene. In fact, all of these aspects of health have much in common. They begin with awareness—you need to recognize that sleep is not a luxury, but a basic component of good health.

Next, you need to commit to spending the time and discipline it takes to get enough sleep, just as you make time to take an after-dinner walk, purchase healthier foods, or floss your teeth. With sleep, this means mentally blocking off certain hours for sleep and then following through on your intention, avoiding accumulation

Repaying a Sleep Debt

Building up a sleep debt is similar to building up a monetary debt in that the less sleep or money you deposit, the bigger the shortfall. However, the debts differ in terms of repayment. While you do have to sleep more than usual to repay a sleep debt, this repayment does not need to be made on a literal one-for-one basis.

- **Short-term.** For example, if you've built up ten hours of sleep debt over a week, several days of getting the sleep you need, plus an additional hour or so per night, should take care of the debt. Then you can return to getting the sleep your body needs (without the additional hour).
- **Long-term.** Similarly, if you've accumulated hundreds or thousands of hours of sleep debt due to a lifetime of bad sleep habits, it won't take you years to repay the debt. Instead, a few

of sleep debt, taking steps to set up an ideal sleep environment (something we'll cover in Chapter 6), and seeking a doctor's help if conventional steps toward good sleep prove insufficient.

This doesn't mean you that you can't have any fun or that you need to beat yourself up if you don't get eight hours of sleep 365 days a year. Just as an occasional slice of chocolate layer cake won't make you obese, staying up a few extra hours for a party or a concert is perfectly acceptable—as long as you make plans to compensate the next day by sleeping in, taking a short afternoon nap, or going to bed earlier.

But over the long haul, you need to make sure you consistently get enough sleep. If you have to get up at 7 A.M. to be at work by nine, this may mean foregoing the late-night talk shows—or taping them for viewing the next evening. If your flight home from a vacation was delayed and you didn't get to bed until 2 A.M., make sure you allow time over the next day or two to catch up on lost sleep.

weeks of getting the sleep you need, plus a bit more, should clear the slate.

You don't have to make up every hour because your body recovers from sleep deprivation by sleeping in a more efficient manner. When you start to catch up on sleep, you initially skip through Stages 1 and 2 more quickly and spend a higher-than-normal percentage of time in deep sleep—the type of sleep most critical for physical and mental recuperation. Once the sleep debt is repaid, the ratios return to their normal levels.

Just as the key to eliminating a monetary debt is to continue paying more than needed each month until your debt is erased, the same is true with sleep. You will know you have paid back your debt when you wake up in the morning feeling refreshed and you are not at all sleepy until you go to bed at night.

Benefits of Sleep

If you're used to treating sleep as a second-class citizen in your life, then you've got some work to do. The only way to erase a sleep debt is to get more sleep. It will take some time to fully recover lost sleep but you will feel the effects quickly. The good news is that people who successfully make the switch from constant sleep debt to regular, sufficient sleep often notice improvements in these areas:

- **Alertness/performance.** Studies show that people who get enough sleep consistently outperform those who do not on driving simulators and reaction time tests. The poor performance of sleep-deprived people is not permanent and improves after getting adequate amounts of sleep. When you're well rested, you feel vigorous throughout the day. You enjoy a good challenge, and when problems arise, you have the energy to solve them instead of procrastinating. Instead of watching the clock at the end of the workday, you're more likely to suddenly discover it's time to go home.

- **Memory, concentration, and creativity.** Getting enough sleep is associated with improved memory and creativity. So instead of wasting time searching for your car keys, you're more likely to come up with a more efficient way of doing your job, tackle a home improvement project, or write a poem to your love.

- **Better health.** Research has shown that short-term sleep debt is associated with minor health problems such as headaches, colds, and stomach discomfort, and that long-term sleep debt is linked to obesity, heart problems, diabetes, and shorter life spans. So it's not surprising that people who start getting sufficient sleep after months or years of sleep debt often see a significant improvement in their overall health.

It's a cliché, but it all comes down to quality of life—whatever your interests and goals, getting enough sleep puts you in a better position to enjoy and achieve them.

Next, we'll look at how and why people sleep differently during the various phases of life.

4

Sleep and Age:
Why Can't I Sleep
Like I Used To?

Of all the factors that affect how a person sleeps, one of the most important is aging. Each stage of life introduces subtle and not-so-subtle changes. Let's take a look at what occurs in each phase.

Childhood

Change is most dramatic during the early years of life; not until the end of adolescence do humans settle into a pattern that remains relatively stable from year to year.

Newborns

Because the biological clock is not yet fully developed at birth, newborns' sleep does not adhere to a twenty-four-hour schedule (or any schedule). Newborns simply sleep a lot; unless they're being fed, changed, or nurtured, they're asleep—from eleven to eighteen hours a day. Sleep occurs in random chunks lasting from a few minutes to several hours, surrounding stretches of wakefulness from one to three hours.

About half of newborns' sleep time is spent in REM sleep. In babies, REM sleep is known as active sleep because they often twitch their arms and legs, smile, or move their bodies about. The other half of sleep time is spent in non-REM (or quiet) sleep, during which the child doesn't move and seems most at rest. A full sleep cycle (from Stage 1 through REM sleep) takes an hour or less, compared to the typical ninety-minute cycle for children and adults.

Infants

At about four weeks, babies' sleep periods start to lengthen. The developing biological clock also begins to exert itself, and infants gradually acquire a more regular sleep/wake cycle. For example, a baby may develop a routine of falling asleep around midnight, waking up for a feeding at about 3 A.M., and then sleeping until dawn.

By six months, most infants begin sleeping through the night and taking naps in the morning and afternoon. Infants typically sleep nine to twelve hours during the night and take thirty-minute to two-hour naps one to four times a day. The number of naps decreases as they reach their first birthday.

Toddlers

After the temporary dip during infancy, sleep time increases again from age one to three, with most toddlers sleeping from twelve to fourteen hours a day. At eighteen months, most toddlers take a single one- to three-hour nap per day. During this phase, toddlers may experience their first frustrations with sleep, such as resistance to bedtime, nighttime awakenings, and nightmares.

Preschoolers

From age three to five, sleep time again drops slightly to eleven to thirteen hours a day. Daytime naps gradually shorten, and by age five, most children no longer nap. As with toddlers, preschoolers may occasionally complain of difficulty falling asleep, waking up during the night, and nightmares. In addition, more serious sleep problems—such as sleepwalking, sleep terrors (screaming while asleep and other physical events), and bed-wetting—may arise.

We'll cover childhood sleep disorders and their treatments in detail in Chapter 17.

Young Children

Between six years and puberty, children's sleep patterns resemble their eventual adult pattern, except that children need more sleep—about ten or eleven hours each night. Nocturnal melatonin production is at its lifetime peak, and children typically have no trouble falling quickly into deep and restorative sleep. Unfortunately, this is the time when demands from the outside world first begin to conflict with the need for sleep. School brings an early wake-up time, homework, and other extracurricular and social activities. Sports, television, video games, and the Internet also compete for sleep time, and youngsters may start to consume caffeinated beverages. As a result, we start to see our first significant divide between how much sleep people need and how much they actually achieve—despite the need for ten hours or more, many young kids get only eight hours or less.

At this stage, the incidence of bed-wetting, sleepwalking, and sleep terrors steadily drops, but nightmares and difficulty falling or staying asleep may persist or develop for the first time in a small percentage of kids. Poor or inadequate sleep can lead to mood swings and behavioral problems such as hyperactivity and an inability to pay attention in class.

Adolescents

Except for infancy, adolescence is the most rapid period of body growth and development. Teens continue to need a lot of sleep (nine or ten hours), but it becomes increasingly hard for them to obtain it. School and social demands increase, and many adolescents take part-time jobs in the evening to earn spending money.

Making matters worse is a biological component. Adolescents' circadian sleep/wake rhythm promotes going to bed late and sleeping late—from about midnight to 9 A.M. or later. But high school typically starts earlier than elementary or middle school, so the morning alarm clock severely truncates sleep. The resulting

41

sleep deprivation means teens often struggle to stay alert and pay attention in class.

A few school districts across the United States have made school start times later—with positive results on sleep and academic performance—but most haven't. In spite of their greater need, teenagers average about seven and a half hours of sleep a day, with many trying to get by on six or less. Exhausted teens often sleep late on weekends to catch up, which throws their body clocks off even more, making it harder to fall asleep on Sunday night.

Although most adolescents do not have difficulty falling and staying asleep when they're tired, a minority may experience sleep disorders more commonly associated with adulthood, such as obstructive sleep apnea, narcolepsy, restless legs syndrome, and circadian rhythm disorders.

Adulthood

From age twenty to sixty, sleep patterns evolve much more slowly than during youth. Large-scale studies have noted a number of consistent trends; as you might expect, good sleep gets harder to achieve over time. Table 4.1 and Figure 4.1 show key data on sleep changes through adulthood:

- **It takes longer to fall sleep.** Sleep researchers refer to how long it takes to fall asleep as sleep latency. The change in sleep latency is small and slow but continual, increasing from an average of about sixteen minutes at age twenty to eighteen minutes at age sixty.
- **You sleep less at night.** Total nighttime sleep decreases from about 7.5 hours at age twenty, to about 7 hours at age forty, to about 6.2 hours at age sixty. The need for sleep remains the same, so many people compensate for the decline in nighttime sleep as they age by taking daytime naps.
- **Stages 1 and 2 sleep increase, while Stages 3 and 4 and REM sleep decrease.** Although you still pass through

TABLE 4.1 Sleep Changes During Adulthood

	Age 20	Age 40	Age 60	Age 70	Age 80
Sleep latency	16 minutes	17 minutes	18 minutes	18.5 minutes	19 minutes
Total sleep time	7.5 hours	7 hours	6.2 hours	6 hours	5.8 hours
Percentage of time in Stage 2 sleep	47	51	53	55	57
Percentage of time in deep sleep	20	15	10	9	7.5
Percentage of time in REM sleep	22	21	20	19	17
Sleep efficiency	95	88	84	82	79

Source: M. Ohayon, et al. "Meta-Analysis of Quantitative Sleep Parameters from Childhood to Old Age in Healthy Individuals: Developing Normative Sleep Values Across the Human Lifespan," *Sleep* 27 (7), 2004: 1255–73.

FIGURE 4.1 Sleep Changes Over Time

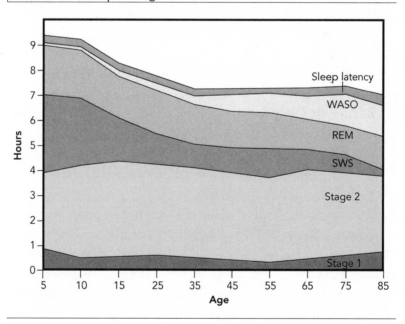

As people age, it takes longer to fall asleep (increased sleep latency), and nighttime awakenings become more frequent (increased wake after sleep onset). In addition, they spend more time in Stage 1 and 2 sleep and less time in deep sleep and REM sleep. REM = rapid eye movement; SWS = slow wave sleep; WASO = wake after sleep onset. Adapted from M. Ohayon, et al., "Meta-Analysis of Quantitative Sleep Parameters from Childhood to Old Age in Healthy Individuals: Developing Normative Sleep Values Across the Human Lifespan," *Sleep* 27 (7), 2004: 1270.

all the sleep stages, you linger longer in Stages 1 and 2. The percentage of time spent in Stage 2 sleep increases 5 to 10 percent every twenty years.

By contrast, you pass more quickly through Stages 3 and 4 (deep sleep) and REM. The percentage of time spent in deep sleep falls by about 50 percent between ages twenty and sixty, and time spent in REM declines by about 9 percent. These changes in sleep stage distribution—which are less severe for women than for men—may be a key reason sleep becomes less restorative over time.

- **Nighttime awakenings increase.** There are several ways to measure the continuity of sleep. One is to count how much time people spend awake after first falling asleep, called wake after sleep onset (WASO). People typically wake up many times for brief periods during the night. This WASO time rises from about eighteen minutes at age twenty to forty-four minutes at age sixty.

Sleep continuity can also be viewed in terms of sleep efficiency, the percentage of time you spend asleep while in bed. In other words, if you're in bed for eight hours but you're only actually asleep for six, your sleep efficiency is 75 percent. As nighttime awakenings become more frequent and last longer, sleep efficiency steadily slips from an average of 95 percent at age twenty to 84 percent at age sixty.

What explains all these changes in sleep that occur with age, even among generally healthy people? We do not yet have a complete understanding of the answer, but it's likely that a number of physiological changes combine to alter the circadian sleep/wake rhythm. We know, for example, that the brain's natural production of the hormone melatonin decreases significantly during adulthood and old age. Similarly, the overnight dip in body temperature becomes less pronounced as we age, and changes in pituitary gland function lead to increased cortisol and decreased growth hormone production. Such changes—and dozens of others—may help explain why older people take longer to fall asleep, get less deep sleep, and awaken more often during the night.

The increase in awakenings with age is also due in part to the increase in medical and sleep disorders over time. Chronic illnesses that cause pain or troubles with breathing can disrupt sleep. Sleep disorders are more likely to emerge during adulthood. Symptoms of narcolepsy may develop during one's teen years, but they often worsen during adulthood. Sleep apnea and other breathing-related problems associated with obesity typically arise in the thirties, forties, and fifties, decades when people tend to put on weight. The frequency of movement disorders such as restless legs syndrome also increases with age. In addition, women's reproductive cycles can affect their sleep over time.

From Sixty On

After age sixty, the sleep trends of adulthood continue. Sleep latency and the percentage of time spent in Stages 1 and 2 sleep increase, while total sleep time, the percentage of time spent in deep sleep and REM, and sleep efficiency all continue to drop.

Doctors used to reassure older people that they needed less sleep than younger people to function well, but sleep experts now know that isn't true. At any age, most adults need seven and a half to eight hours of sleep a day to function at their best. Because of the trends we've identified, older people often have trouble attaining this much sleep, especially at night. Not surprisingly, the older we get, the more likely we are to supplement nighttime sleep with daytime naps.

The older one gets, the more overall health is directly linked to sleep quantity and quality. Those with severe or multiple health problems may experience major difficulties. For example, sleep problems are prominent in elderly people who develop Alzheimer's disease or other forms of dementia, which are often associated with insomnia, nightmares, wandering, physical aggression, loud screaming and talking, or calling for help. The sleep of

Reproductive Cycles and Sleep

Different aspects of women's reproductive cycles can greatly influence sleep. For example, during the first trimester of pregnancy, many women are tired all the time and may log an extra two hours of sleep a night if their schedules permit. As pregnancy continues, hormonal and anatomical changes reduce sleep efficiency so that less of a woman's time in bed is actually spent sleeping. As a result, fatigue increases.

The postpartum period usually brings dramatic sleepiness and fatigue because the mother's ability to sleep efficiently has not returned to normal, because she is at the mercy of her newborn's rapidly cycling shifts between sleeping and waking, and because breast-feeding promotes sleepiness. Researchers are probing whether sleep disturbances during pregnancy may contribute to postpartum depression and compromise the general physical and mental well-being of new mothers.

partners and other caregivers of people with these illnesses often suffers as well.

The Big Picture

Looking at the sleep story from the womb to the tomb, we've focused on the steady decline in our ability to sleep well and the increase in the various disorders that can arise during different life stages. Although this is an accurate description of the trends that can occur with aging, it doesn't mean that every individual is destined to experience all of what's described in this chapter. A few key points about aging and sleep deserve mention:

- **It's possible to get enough sleep.** From childhood through old age, we see a gap between how much sleep people need and how much they actually get. Note that

Women who aren't pregnant also may experience monthly shifts in sleep habits. During the second phase of the menstrual cycle, between ovulation and the next menses, some women fall asleep and enter REM sleep more quickly than usual. A few experience extreme sleepiness. Investigators are studying the relationship between such sleep alterations, cyclic changes in body temperature, and levels of the hormone progesterone to see whether these physiological patterns also correlate with premenstrual mood changes.

Finally, during menopause, many women experience hot flashes that can interrupt sleep, sometimes leading to chronic insomnia. Therapies directed at reducing menopause symptoms can improve sleep (see Chapter 9).

much of this is a product of modern life, not defects in the body's design. Before the invention of the lightbulb in the nineteenth century, adults typically slept eight or nine hours a night. If you're healthy and set aside sufficient time for sleep, there's no reason you can't get most or all of the sleep your body needs.

- **Some decline is natural.** As we've seen, increasing age is associated with decreases in sleep latency and total sleep time and increases in nighttime awakenings. While this sounds discouraging, this information can also be empowering; these changes are perfectly normal and nothing to panic about. Instead, let them be your cue to start putting some extra effort into achieving optimal sleep.
- **How much things change is health–dependent.** While people with health problems often experience major difficulties sleeping as they age, the flip side is that healthy

people usually do not. If you maintain good health through a regular exercise regimen, eating a balanced diet, and making good sleep habits a priority, you're likely to experience only minor sleep changes as you age. It may take a few more minutes to fall asleep at age sixty than it did at age twenty, and you may get up a couple of times during the night, but overall you can still feel like the same old you.

Next, we'll look some common sleep myths.

CHAPTER 5

Sleep Myths and Facts

Even with all the facts you've learned so far, I'm sure you still have some nagging doubts about the many stories you've heard about how others sleep, things you can do to get better sleep, and what sleep really does for you. Many of these tales are left over from before researchers began to study and understand sleep. Before we address how to improve your sleep habits, let's clear up some of the most common sleep myths.

You Need Less Sleep as You Get Older

As children, many of us had grandparents who always seemed to be up at the crack of dawn, cleaning the house and making a glorious breakfast. So it seemed as if older people didn't need as much sleep as other adults.

This memory overlooks a couple of things: Grandma and Grandpa were probably in bed by 9 P.M., and they often disappeared in the early afternoon to take a nap. In truth, older people need just as much as sleep as younger adults. They may have trouble getting it because they wake up more frequently during the night, but total sleep need does not decrease much with age.

Alcohol Helps You Sleep Better

As we will discuss in Chapter 6, alcohol is not an effective sleep aid. Its sedative effect may make you fall asleep faster, but it has a harmful effect on sleep quality that far outweighs this benefit. When alcohol is in your body, you get less of the deep sleep you need to wake up feeling refreshed, you're more likely to wake up during the night, and you're more likely to snore and experience other nocturnal breathing problems.

Snoring Is Annoying but Harmless

There's no doubt that snoring is annoying. In some cases it is harmless, but in others it's a sign of obstructive sleep apnea, a sleep disorder characterized by pauses in breathing that prevent air from flowing into or out of a sleeping person's airways. As we will see in Chapter 11, sleep apnea increases a person's risk of heart disease and causes severe daytime sleepiness. Snorers who temporarily stop breathing during the night or experience severe daytime sleepiness should consult a physician.

There's Something Wrong If You Don't Remember Your Dreams

Everybody dreams, but some people remember them and some don't. Not being able to recall your dreams is perfectly normal and has no negative health effects. Whether or not you remember your dreams is determined by when you wake up in relation to having those dreams. If you wake up during or just after a dream, you're likely to remember it; otherwise, you won't. It's just a matter of timing and has no bearing on sleep quality.

If you've never had much luck remembering your dreams but would like to, a few techniques can help. The trick is to try to recall them the moment you wake up—letting time pass seems to function as an erase button on your mental VCR, especially if you fall back asleep. Keep a pen and pad on your nightstand and jot down notes about your dreams when you wake up, whether it's at your normal wake-up time or after waking during the night. If you do this every night for a week, there's a good chance you'll start regularly recalling your dreams.

I Can Get by Fine on Five or Six Hours of Sleep

It's true that a small percentage of people are short sleepers who only need five or six hours of sleep per night. However, sometimes it seems as if two-thirds of the population believe they belong to this select group.

The overwhelming majority of people need seven to nine hours a night, so the chances are relatively small that any particular individual is truly a short sleeper. To calculate your sleep need, follow the instructions in Chapter 3.

If you need eight hours a night but only get six, you can usually carry on for a day or two. After a few days, you'll start to show signs of sleep deprivation, such as daytime drowsiness, irritability, and decreased productivity, and you'll also place yourself at a higher risk for safety problems at work and behind the wheel.

You Can Learn to Get by on Less Sleep

Unfortunately, there's no way to train the body to reduce its sleep need. Studies on chronic partial sleep deprivation, restricting people to only four or five hours of sleep for several weeks, found that people continue to get sleepier and their performance becomes more impaired the longer the study goes on. There is no plateau or limit to how sleepy and impaired they get. To meet a job deadline or study for a final exam you may be able to function on less sleep, but you will feel more tired, work less efficiently, and get less done.

Insomniacs Barely Sleep at All

People with insomnia often announce in the morning that they "didn't sleep at all last night." Although it may have seemed this way, failing to get any sleep is extremely unlikely. Even in severe cases, people with insomnia typically get a few hours of sleep per night. We all tend to be poor judges of how long it takes us to fall asleep and how long we've slept. Everyone has had the experience of intending to fall asleep for a few minutes and waking up several hours later, unaware of how much time has passed. This is because we don't experience the passing of time while asleep. There is a small group of people who are convinced they get no sleep at all each night—until we bring them into the sleep laboratory and show them that although they claimed to lie awake all night, they actually slept for seven hours.

Falling Asleep During the Day Is a Sign of Laziness

Falling asleep during daytime hours is not a character defect; it's a sign of physiological need. Lazy people may fritter away their time at unproductive or pointless tasks, but they don't necessarily have trouble staying awake in the daytime.

Sleeping during the day is a sign of sleep deprivation. This can be self-induced (that is, from staying up late), or it may result from poor sleep hygiene; insomnia; sleep apnea, narcolepsy, or another sleep disorder; or an underlying illness. It can also be a side effect of a medication.

Listening to Self-Help Recordings While You Sleep Can Help You Learn

Although a multitude of tapes and CDs are available on the Internet purporting to help people improve themselves (such as learn a language, lose weight, or quit smoking) while they sleep, I've yet to see any solid research showing they're effective. What sometimes confuses this issue is that there is abundant evidence that a good night's rest can improve test performance compared to a night of sleep deprivation. Sleep does play a role in learning, but first you need to be awake while you're taking in new information.

Napping Is a Bad Habit

Napping is a complex issue—depending on the situation, a nap can be either helpful or harmful. The major factor to consider is what effect a nap will have on your main sleep block. If it's likely to curtail it, then napping is inadvisable, since ideally you want the main sleep period to be as long as possible. If a nap is unlikely to affect the main sleep block, then it's perfectly okay.

"Bad" naps come up most often in the context of people with chronic insomnia. These people often get less than six hours of sleep at night, leading them to feel sleepy during the day. Giving in and taking a nap—especially a long one—only perpetuates the cycle of nighttime insomnia and daytime sleepiness. In such cases, the individual needs to pinpoint the source of the insomnia and address it (see Chapters 8 and 9).

The timing of a nap can also affect its desirability. If you keep traditional hours, it's generally a bad idea to nap in the evening, since this makes it harder to fall asleep at night. Unless your safety is in danger and you need the nap to stay awake for the next few hours, you're usually better off toughing it out until your regular bedtime.

In most other situations, though, naps are beneficial. For example, if you don't have insomnia but experience an occasional night of short sleep (from work stress, noisy neighbors, child care demands, and so on), then a nap is a great way to replace your lost sleep. Many people whose sleep is curtailed by the morning alarm clock routinely squeeze in a short afternoon nap, and this is healthy. Naps are also a lifesaver for shift workers, due to the sleep deprivation that frequently accompanies working at night (see Chapter 16).

It's Possible to Get Too Much Sleep

You've probably heard people say that if they sleep too much they feel tired when they wake up. This is a misconception. First, you can't get more sleep than your body needs. The homeostatic drive to sleep wears off as you sleep and stops exerting its pressure. In the morning, the circadian cycle is in its alert phase, not its sleep phase. So if you continue to sleep, it's because you need more sleep.

Second, the grogginess that some people report with longer sleep isn't due to the extended sleep. Most often, people extend their sleep because they've been depriving themselves for several nights. A single night of extended sleep does not make up all of the sleep debt, so when they wake up, they're still sleep deprived and as a result don't feel refreshed.

Finally, if you extend your sleep into the afternoon you may wake up at a time on your circadian clock when it's natural to be sleepy, which may contribute to that groggy feeling.

Don't let fear of feeling bad keep you from getting enough sleep. Listen to your body; it will tell you whether or not you need more sleep. If you're sleepy, you need more sleep.

How I Sleep Doesn't Affect the Rest of My Health

More and more evidence is accumulating showing that overall health is very much tied to sleep quality and quantity. Specific sleep disorders, such as sleep apnea, can cause hypertension and heart disease. Mood and mental health are affected by sleep. Sleep deprivation is linked to the development of obesity, diabetes, and heart disease and can even affect your life span. So give sleep its due.

Next, let's look at the basics of getting a good night's sleep.

CHAPTER 6

How to Get a Good Night's Sleep: A Six-Step Plan

Thanks to technology, with the push of a button you can summon a movie on your television, speed-dial a friend's cell phone, or ensure that fresh coffee awaits you in the morning. No such button instantly puts you to sleep and wakes you up feeling refreshed, but there are numerous measures you can take that will give you the best chance possible of getting a good night's sleep. In the sleep improvement plan that follows, I've divided these measures into six general categories:

- Recognizing the importance of sleep
- Adopting a healthy lifestyle
- Maintaining good sleep habits
- Creating the optimal sleep environment
- Watching out for sleep saboteurs
- Seeking help for persistent sleep problems

Recognize the Importance of Sleep

We've covered this point in previous chapters, but I'll say it one more time: *Sleep is essential to good health, so you need to block out sufficient time to get the sleep your body needs.* If your body requires eight hours of sleep each night and you only set aside six or seven, you won't receive the full benefit of any other changes you make. Failing to take this first step is the sleep equivalent of drawing the Do Not Pass Go card in Monopoly.

Adopt a Healthy Lifestyle

We saw in Chapter 3 how good sleep promotes good health. The reverse is also true. Good health habits—such as exercising regularly, maintaining a healthy diet, and avoiding cigarettes and excessive alcohol—set the stage for good sleep.

- **Exercise regularly.** Exercise is extremely important to healthy living. It improves fitness, prevents illness, and increases longevity. Exercise also improves sleep. Research has repeatedly shown that exercise provides three critical benefits: you fall asleep faster, attain a higher percentage of deep sleep, and awaken less often during the night.

  Exercise seems to be of particular benefit to older people. A Duke University study found that physically fit older men fall asleep in less than half the time it takes for sedentary men, and they wake up less often during the night. Researchers from the University of Washington found that older men and women who reported sleeping normally could still increase the amount of time they spent in deep sleep if they engaged in aerobic activity.

  You don't have to run marathons or play full-court basketball to earn exercise's benefits. Most of the advantages come from temporarily elevating your heart rate for twenty to thirty minutes three or more times a week. Brisk

Why Exercise Enhances Sleep

The benefit of regular exercise to people who have trouble sleeping probably occurs because it reduces stress and anxiety, factors that impede sleep. A good workout leaves you feeling relaxed and in a good mood, so later on you're more likely to fall asleep and stay asleep.

The underlying mechanism for exercise's sleep-enhancing effect has not been conclusively determined. One theory is that regular exercise and the subsequent increase in physical fitness that results boosts the brain's production of serotonin, a chemical that promotes sleep.

Another theory centers on body temperature change, also known as thermoregulation. Exercise temporarily heats up your body and brain. Once you're done exercising, you cool down, and this cooling-down process may better prepare your body for sleep.

Exercise also has an effect on your biological clock. Researchers have been able to shift subjects' biological clocks with properly timed exercise. They theorize that daytime exercise helps lock your circadian rhythm of sleep and wakefulness into a consistent twenty-four-hour pattern, ensuring that you're ready to fall asleep when bedtime arrives.

walking, jogging, bicycling, swimming, and aerobics all accomplish this. Find the activity you enjoy most and incorporate regular workouts into your life.

One important caveat here is that you should not exercise too close to bedtime because this is a stimulating activity that can make it harder to fall asleep. If you finish exercising at least two hours before bedtime, you'll eliminate this risk.

- **Maintain a healthy diet.** While the pros and cons of particular foods may seem to change with the latest headlines, the overall benefits of consuming a healthy diet and avoiding obesity are not in dispute. It may be easier said than done, but you should strive to maintain a high-fiber, low-fat diet that's rich in fruits, vegetables, and whole grains. Such a diet helps keep your cholesterol, blood pressure, and weight down, lowering your risk for cardiovascular problems, diabetes, and other severe health problems associated with poorer sleep. There's no need to starve yourself—just always be conscious of what and how much you eat. If you have questions about how much of which foods you should have (it can be confusing), consult a nutritionist or your primary care physician.

- **Don't drink to excess or smoke.** The negative long-term health effects of alcohol abuse (liver disease, depression, and so on) and smoking (such as increased risk for cancer and cardiovascular disease) are well known. Both also have immediate deleterious effects on sleep, as you'll see later in this chapter. If you smoke or have a problem with alcohol, talk to your doctor about finding a strategy or program that will help you quit.

Maintain Good Sleep Habits

The tips in this section and the next two fall under what is often called *sleep hygiene*. The idea is that just as there are things you do for your personal and dental hygiene, following certain steps will lead to healthy sleep.

- **Keep a regular sleep/wake schedule.** As noted in Chapter 2, a regular sleep schedule keeps the circadian cycle synchronized by conditioning the body to expect specific sleep and wake-up times. Once you've determined how much sleep you need, you need to set up a sleep schedule and adhere to it as much as possible. The exact hours you choose will depend on your work schedule and commuting pattern, as well as your tendency to be a lark or an owl. But whatever works for you, the important thing is to stick with it seven days a week. If you must deviate from this schedule on weekends, try to limit the change in wake-up time to a maximum of an hour.

In addition to regular sleep and wake times, aim to do other significant activities—such as meals and exercise sessions—at consistent times. If you have dinner at six on Monday, at nine on Tuesday, and at eight on Wednesday, you send your body conflicting messages about when it should expect sleep to begin.

- **Develop a presleep routine.** Similarly, you should develop a routine for the hours leading up to bedtime—you can't expect to walk in the door, hop into bed, and fall asleep. Instead, start by setting aside fifteen to twenty minutes to resolve any mundane matters that might otherwise be on your mind if left undone when you go to bed (unwashed dishes, plans for the next day, responding to personal e-mail, and so on). Then try to wind down from the day with a nonstrenuous activity, such as reading, watching television, or listening to music. Many people find an evening shower or bath helps them relax.

  If you often find yourself dwelling on personal problems while in bed, it may be helpful to set them aside beforehand with a writing exercise. Write your concerns down on a pad of paper or some index cards and put them to one side. Then tell yourself you will work on them tomorrow. This way you won't have to spend time dwelling on them while you try to sleep. (If new worries or ideas often arise when you're already in bed, and fear of forgetting them keeps you awake, keep the pad near your bed so you can jot down a quick note and quickly return to falling sleep.)

  Yet another possibility is to use the presleep time to practice any stress management techniques you've learned, such as relaxation exercises, meditation, and biofeedback. We'll discuss these techniques in greater depth when we cover insomnia treatments in Chapter 8.

Obviously, there are many options for the hours before bedtime—the important thing is to identify activities you enjoy doing that relax you and reduce stress, and then order them in a way that's likely to make you ready for sleep.

- **Reserve the bedroom for sleep and intimacy.** You want your body to associate your bed with sleep as much as possible, so the sight and feel of your bed subconsciously sends a message to your brain that "sleep is on the way." For this reason, it's advisable to reserve the bedroom for two activities—sleep and sex. Even though it's comfortable in bed, resist the impulse to watch television, balance your checkbook, make phone calls, eat a snack, and so on.

- **Avoid frequent naps.** Short naps can be beneficial if you're sleep deprived and need an alertness boost; we'll discuss smart napping strategies in Chapter 16 on challenging sleep situations. But if you routinely have trouble falling asleep at night, you generally want to confine sleep to one long nighttime segment.

  The rationale behind this policy is that the homeostatic drive for sleep increases the longer you've been awake. If you nap at 7 P.M., you cut the potential number of consecutive hours awake before nighttime sleep from sixteen or so down to about four—a reduction that can make it hard to fall asleep. In the long run, giving in to the urge to nap in the evening only perpetuates the cycle of poor nighttime sleep and daytime sleepiness.

- **If you can't sleep, get out of bed.** Bed is for sleep, not frustration. When you have trouble falling asleep, don't spend hours lying in bed, tossing and turning and getting exasperated. Twenty or thirty minutes is a good cutoff point; if you're not asleep by then, get up and do something soothing—such as reading or drinking milk or herbal tea. This practice prevents you from perceiving the bed as a battleground where you're likely to become agitated and have problems sleeping. Be sure not to fill this time with stimulating activities that would interfere with sleep, such as paying bills, cleaning, or playing computer games. When you start to feel sleepy, return to bed and go to sleep.

Create the Optimal Sleep Environment

You want every element of your bedroom to encourage sleep. Evaluate the room and try to identify what might be getting in the way of a good night's sleep.

- **Control bedroom noise.** Nothing is more annoying than drifting into sleep, only to be jolted awake by the sound of a dog barking or a car stereo. Take steps to reduce or disguise noises that can interfere with sleep. Ear plugs are remarkably effective in blocking out unwanted noise. No need to get fancy—just pick up a box of silicone or foam earplugs for a few dollars at your local drugstore. You can also better soundproof your room by installing double-paned windows and decorating with heavy curtains and rugs, which absorb sounds. If you're frequently awakened by unwanted calls or visitors, learn how to disconnect your phone and doorbell at night.

  Finally, some people find it beneficial to use an appliance that produces a steady "white noise" to obscure outside sounds. You can use an ordinary fan or purchase a white noise device designed specifically to provide this kind of steady hum.

- **Block out light.** As we've seen, light signals the biological clock in the brain that it's time to wake up. The darker it is, the better, so use thick curtains, curtain liners, or blackout shades to ensure that light does not come through the windows. Also, check for light sources inside the room. Most electronic devices have lighted displays that can produce enough light to disturb sleep if not covered up. If you're still aware of light after trying to address external and internal sources, wear eye shades.

- **Keep it cool and well ventilated.** The ideal temperature for sleep is a matter of personal preference. In general, you should make sure it's not too hot and that air circulates freely so you don't feel that your room is stuffy. If you're often congested, you may wish to run a humidifier.

  Also, be aware that your body temperature drops during the overnight hours. Have an additional blanket or a sweatshirt available if you wake up feeling chilly.

- **Hide the clock.** For some people, the sight of the time can be disconcerting, since it serves as a taunting reminder that you're awake, both when you're trying to fall asleep and when you wake up during the night. If this applies to you, turn the alarm clock around or cover it up before you go to sleep.

- **Make your bed comfortable.** You need a bed you like using, so put some effort into finding the comfort, firmness, and design that suit you. If you've had the same mattress for more than a decade, it's worthwhile spending an hour or two testing mattresses and buying one that feels right. Then put similar energy into finding comfortable pajamas, blankets, and pillows.

Watch Out for Sleep Saboteurs

A final aspect of good sleep hygiene is awareness of how beverages and other substances can interfere with sleep.

- **Limit caffeine.** As you no doubt know from experience, caffeine boosts alertness. It does this by blocking the effect of adenosine, a chemical produced by neurons in the brain that promotes sleep. (Such brain chemicals are known as neurotransmitters.) As a result, caffeine lengthens the time it takes to fall asleep and reduces the amount of deep sleep you get. In addition, caffeine is a diuretic, meaning it can further disrupt sleep by increasing the need to urinate during the night.

Individuals vary greatly in their sensitivity to caffeine; you may need to experiment to determine your own threshold. Caffeine's half-life—the time it takes for half of it to clear your system—is three to five hours, so it's still active in your body long after you've had your last caffeinated drink of the day. Avoid heavy overall intake (more than two or three cups of coffee, tea, or caffeinated soda a day) and curtail consumption after 5 or 6 P.M. If you try this and still have trouble sleeping, you may benefit from even stricter limits, such as cutting down to one cup before 2 P.M. or even foregoing caffeine altogether.

Two final caffeine points: Be aware that in addition to beverages, chocolate and certain cold medications (check the label) can contain significant amounts of caffeine. Also, your body can become dependent on caffeine, so if you're a heavy consumer cut back gradually or you may experience headaches, irritability, and fatigue.

- **Use alcohol cautiously.** In the sleep world, alcohol is the wolf in sheep's clothing; a nightcap may help you drop off, but this benefit is more than offset by the poor-quality sleep that ensues.

Alcohol tends to decrease sleep latency, meaning that you fall asleep quicker. However, it's a rocky road once you do nod off: Deep sleep (Stages 3 and 4) and REM sleep are both sharply reduced, so most of what you get is of the less refreshing Stage 1 or 2 variety, and you're likely to wake up more during the latter half of the night because decreasing alcohol levels fragment sleep. The fact that alcohol is also a diuretic further adds to sleep disruption, since you may have to get up to go to the bathroom. Finally, because alcohol relaxes throat muscles and interferes with brain control mechanisms, it can worsen snoring and other nocturnal breathing problems, sometimes to a dangerous extent.

For all these reasons, you're liable to feel worn out when the alarm goes off if you drink to help yourself fall asleep. To prevent alcohol from interfering with sleep, limit yourself to one or two drinks a day, and finish drinking at least three hours before bedtime. The body metabolizes alcohol faster than caffeine, so your cutoff point can be a few hours closer to bedtime.

- **Stop smoking or chewing tobacco.** Nicotine is a central nervous system stimulant that speeds your heart rate, raises blood pressure, and incites fast brain wave activity that interferes with sleep. In people addicted to nicotine, a few hours without it is enough to induce withdrawal symptoms; the craving can then wake them up at night.

  People who kick the habit fall asleep more quickly and wake less often during the night. Sleep disturbances and daytime fatigue may occur during the initial withdrawal period, but even during this time, many former users report improvements in sleep. Quitting also offers a host of other health benefits, including a lower risk for cancer, heart disease, and stroke.

- **Find the right balance of fluids.** Beverages with caffeine and alcohol are a bad idea before bed, but that doesn't mean you should curtail all fluid intake. You want to find the right balance—if you drink too much liquid in the evening, you may wake up to use the bathroom. On the other hand, if you eliminate liquids altogether for several hours before bedtime, you're liable to become dehydrated during the night and wake up dry and thirsty. Use common sense. If you wake up often to go to the bathroom, cut back on evening fluids. If you're often thirsty at night, have something to drink before bedtime.

- **Avoid foods that give you heartburn.** What you eat, as well as how much and when, can affect sleep. Heartburn is the most common problem; lying down makes it worse, and it can wake you up during the night. General indigestion and feeling bloated also can impede sleep.

The goal is to have the stomach's most difficult digestive work wrapped up long before you go to bed. Avoid fatty and spicy foods that can give you indigestion, don't eat too much, and make sure to allow several hours between dinner and bedtime. If you continue to have heartburn, elevate the head of your bed to prevent the reflux of acidic stomach contents while you are sleeping. Just using extra pillows isn't enough. You can also ask your doctor whether you're likely to benefit from heartburn medication.

At the same time, you don't want to go to bed hungry and have your stomach growling. If you find this is often the case, have a light snack an hour or two before bedtime.

Seek Help for Persistent Sleep Problems

All the tips in this chapter are basics that everyone who has trouble sleeping should try. As you read it, perhaps you found one or more flaws in your lifestyle and sleep regimen. If so, there's a good chance that fixing the problems will lead to significantly improved sleep. Maybe you'll even pronounce yourself cured and have no need to read the rest of the book.

Of course, this chapter will not be a panacea for everyone. You may already follow these guidelines, or you may make some important changes but fail to realize major improvements. If these simple steps don't improve your sleep, you should consult your physician or a sleep specialist. Much can still be done, including identifying a sleep disorder. And keep reading—there are numerous treatment options we've yet to discuss, one of which may be the key to improving your sleep.

That concludes our first section. In Part II, we'll look at specific sleep disorders and their treatments, beginning with a chapter on how you can narrow down the source of your sleep problem.

PART 11

Sleep Disorders and Their Treatments

CHAPTER 7

Signs of a Sleep Problem

When I see a patient for the first time, one of the first questions I ask is, "What is the problem with your sleep?" Responses fall into five general categories:

- I can't fall asleep.
- I can't stay awake.
- I can't get up in the morning.
- I do strange things in my sleep.
- I can't sleep because of my partner.

How would you answer this question? Each complaint can be caused by one of several disorders, so your response is just the start of the search for the cause of your sleep difficulty. But your initial response will help you narrow down what the culprit is likely to be. If you find yourself saying, "That really sounds like me" as you read the description for a certain category, feel free to skip ahead to the chapters on the relevant disorders.

I Can't Fall Asleep

People use this phrase to describe a number of problems, all of which share the feature of an inability to get to sleep in a desired length of time. The difficulty can occur when first getting into bed, after waking up in the middle of the night, or in the early-morning hours.

I Can't Get to Sleep

For many people, the primary problem is sleep latency—they have difficulty falling asleep. Instead, they toss and turn as the minutes, and even hours, go by. Once this pattern has been established, they may try ill-advised measures to break it, such as distracting themselves with television or drinking a nightcap before bed. Often they start to feel anxious before bedtime, fearing they won't be able to fall asleep. They may delay going to bed for several hours, convinced there's no chance they'll fall asleep. Eventually, they do fall asleep from exhaustion, but they may end up getting only a few hours of sleep before it's time to get up in the morning. The next night, the scenario repeats.

Problems with sleep latency are most often due to one of the following:

- **Sleep onset insomnia (Chapter 8).** People who can't fall asleep may have a type of insomnia that stems from a problem known as overactivation. In other words, activity within the brain does not slow down enough to allow them to make the transition from wakefulness to sleep. Sometimes this is triggered by a disturbing event like a death in the family or the loss of a job, but frequently there is no specific event. Often, the initial sleep difficulty is compounded by anxiety that becomes self-perpetuating—insomnia causes anxiety about sleep, which in turn causes more insomnia. As they enter the bedroom, these people start to worry about whether or not they will fall asleep, which causes them to become more alert. This makes it harder to fall asleep, which further increases their concern, boosting alertness, and so on.

- **Delayed sleep phase disorder (Chapter 15).** A malfunctioning biological clock is another potential obstacle to falling asleep. With the circadian rhythm disorder known as delayed sleep phase disorder, the sleep/wake rhythm is shifted several hours later than it should be. So instead of feeling sleepiest from 11 P.M. to 7 A.M., a person's natural sleep block might be from 3 A.M. to 11 A.M. At midnight, the body still reacts as if it's early in the evening, a time characterized by alertness. This isn't a problem for people whose schedule can accommodate sleeping late, but it is for those who have to be at work or school by 8 A.M.

- **Shift work (Chapter 16).** People who work at night often have trouble falling sleep. Their problems may occur in the morning following a night shift or at night after finishing a stretch of night shifts. Shift workers are often perplexed when they find that after spending all night fighting to stay awake, they can't fall asleep when they finally get home. Here, too, the problem stems from a disrupted circadian rhythm, since these workers frequently must try to sleep at times when their bodies are geared for wakefulness.

- **Restless legs syndrome (Chapter 12).** This sleep disorder causes people to experience unpleasant "creepy crawly" sensations in their legs (and sometimes arms) when they are sitting still or lying down, and they're compelled to move the affected limbs. These feelings occur in the evening, shortly before or after a person gets into bed. Obviously, it's hard to fall asleep if you can't keep still.

- **Paradoxical insomnia.** Individuals' perceptions of how long it takes them to fall asleep and the number of times they wake up are often wildly inaccurate. Paradoxical insomnia is rooted in this misperception. Some people who actually sleep quite well are convinced they hardly sleep at all. These people report poor-quality, nonrefreshing sleep and daytime tiredness. They frequently report not sleeping even a minute for several nights at a time. But when their sleep is measured accurately in a sleep laboratory, they actually get a full night of sleep. For people with this problem, recognizing that they get enough sleep may be all the treatment that's needed.

- **Other medical disorders (Chapter 19).** Health problems that most commonly make it hard to fall asleep include gastroesophageal reflux disease (GERD), hyperthyroidism, chronic pain, and breathing disorders such as emphysema.

I Can't Stay Asleep

Sometimes the biggest problem is repeated awakenings, a phenomenon known as sleep fragmentation. People with this complaint may fall asleep with relative ease at bedtime but wake up an hour or so later. This pattern repeats through the night, so the overnight hours are punctuated by a series of dispiriting clock readings: 1:35, 2:21, 3:06, 4:20, 5:38, and so on. Insufficient sleep leads to daytime fatigue.

Difficulty getting back to sleep can be due to the following:

- **Sleep maintenance insomnia (Chapter 8).** It's not unusual to wake up a few times during the night. Everyone does so briefly, but healthy sleepers fall back asleep so quickly that they have no memory of the few seconds they were awake. It becomes an issue when the person stays awake long enough to become aware that he or she is awake. The individual's brain responds to temporarily waking up as if it's really time to rise and shine—a type of overactivation that researchers refer to as hyperarousal. This can start the same process as in those who have difficulty getting to sleep initially. Once awake, they toss and turn and get frustrated at being awake.
- **Shift work (Chapter 16).** Many shift workers coming off a night shift manage to fall asleep at 8 or 9 A.M. But the challenge of staying asleep during the daytime—when

circadian rhythms are promoting alertness—often proves insurmountable, and they wake up a few hours later. From then on, it's common for people to sleep only in short stretches or to be unable to fall back to sleep.

- **Other medical disorders (Chapter 19).** Medical disorders that fragment sleep can cause problems staying asleep. These include kidney disease, depression, and heart failure, as well as sleep fragmentation disorders such as sleep apnea and periodic limb movements of sleep.

I Wake Up Early in the Morning

Waking up at 4 or 5 A.M. and being unable to get back to sleep can be as troubling as having difficulty falling asleep at bedtime. As a result of the truncated sleep, the person does not feel rested and is tired during the day.

Trouble with early-morning awakening can be due to the following:

- **Sleep maintenance insomnia (Chapter 8).** This is the same problem described in the previous section, except that now there is only one early awakening, and the person never gets back to sleep. The awakening triggers the arousal/ alerting response, leaving the person unable to relax enough to return to sleep.
- **Advanced sleep phase disorder (Chapter 15).** In this circadian rhythm disorder, the sleep/wake rhythm is shifted earlier, so that a person's natural sleep block may be from 8 P.M. until 4 A.M. The individual may find it disturbing to have to go to bed so early and then to be fully awake at an hour when nearly everyone else is still asleep. Again, this is only a problem if the person is unable or unwilling to follow this pattern. Advancing of the circadian rhythm seems to be a property of aging, so it's often elderly people who report this problem.
- **Depression (Chapter 19).** Along with making it hard to fall asleep at night, depression is often associated with early-morning awakenings.

- **Other medical disorders (Chapter 19).** Medical disorders that cause sleep fragmentation, such as heart failure or chronic obstructive pulmonary disease (COPD), can cause early wake-ups. The early-morning pain and stiffness associated with arthritis can also cause this problem.

I Can't Stay Awake

It's normal to feel some mild drowsiness at times during the day, especially during the afternoon. Some people, however, experience daytime drowsiness so severe that they battle—often unsuccessfully—to stay awake. Researchers refer to this phenomenon as excessive daytime sleepiness (EDS). This problem can make getting through the day an epic struggle, and it may lead to poor work performance, automobile accidents, and marital problems. People with EDS may nod off at quiet moments (during a dimly lit meeting or while watching television) or even during not-so-quiet moments (while eating lunch, having a conversation, or driving a car). They frequently underestimate how sleepy they are until prodded to seek medical help by a spouse, friend, or coworker who is frustrated with their sleeping on the job.

Excessive daytime sleepiness can be caused by the following:

- **Narcolepsy (Chapter 13).** Narcolepsy is a neurological disorder in which the brain sends sleep-inducing signals at unpredictable and inappropriate times. Following a wave of extreme sleepiness, people with the disorder may unexpectedly fall asleep. They may also experience a sudden, temporary loss of muscle tone, which causes paralysis of the head or body while the person remains awake and conscious.
- **Sleep apnea (Chapter 11).** People with the breathing disorder known as sleep apnea don't usually have trouble falling asleep at bedtime. Once asleep, though, muscles in the throat relax excessively, collapsing the airway. Breathing is temporarily blocked, sending an emergency signal to the

brain that wakes them up, so they can open their airway and resume breathing. Although sleep is frequently interrupted —sometimes as often as every thirty seconds—their perception of how often they wake up varies, and they are often unaware that sleep apnea is severely fragmenting their sleep. The repeated awakenings cause sleep deprivation, making daytime sleepiness the primary complaint.

- **Periodic limb movement disorder (PLMD) (Chapter 12).** This sleep disorder causes frequent jerking movements of the legs and arms during sleep, which wake a person up. It's related to restless legs syndrome; most people with RLS have PLMD as well, but patients with PLMD often do not have RLS. The combination can cause people both to wake up and to have difficulty getting back to sleep. As with sleep apnea, these disorders can diminish sleep quality to the point that it becomes hard to stay awake during the day.
- **Shift work (Chapter 16).** People who work through the overnight hours often have difficulty staying awake on the job, especially if they sit while working. Days off can also be marred by EDS, since they may be so sleep deprived from working at night and from disruptions of the sleep/wake rhythm that they can't stay awake during leisure time.
- **Advanced sleep phase disorder (Chapter 15).** With this circadian rhythm disorder, the sleep/wake rhythm runs several hours ahead of schedule, prompting strong feelings of sleepiness in the early evening.
- **Other medical disorders (Chapter 19).** Health problems associated with difficulty staying awake include hypothyroidism, neuromuscular diseases, and any medical disorder that fragments sleep.

I Can't Get Up in the Morning

For some people, the worst moment of the day is the second the alarm starts beeping in the morning. They emerge in a daze, searching for the snooze button or turning the alarm off altogether. Once out of bed, it may take an hour or more to fully emerge from the fog. The problem here is what researchers refer to as excessive sleep inertia—difficulty making the transition from sleep to wakefulness.

Sleep inertia may be due to the following:

- **Sleep apnea (Chapter 11).** Most people with sleep apnea are entirely unaware of the interruptions in their sleep. They perceive being asleep for seven or eight consecutive hours, but their sleep is so severely disrupted that it fails to refresh them, and the morning alarm finds them exhausted.
- **Delayed sleep phase disorder (Chapter 15).** People with this disorder—in which the natural sleep block is delayed by several hours—don't feel sleepy at the traditional bedtime, so they may stay up very late. Then the morning alarm goes off at what feels like the middle of the night, often rousing them from deep sleep.
- **Other medical disorders (Chapter 19).** Heart failure and kidney disease are among the health problems associated with difficulty waking up. Medications that can cause drowsiness, such as those prescribed for anxiety and other mood disorders, can make it hard to get up. People suffering from depression don't have trouble waking up but their emotional state can make it difficult for them to get motivated to get out of bed and face the day.

I Do Strange Things in My Sleep

For people in this category, sleep is full of surprises. They may wake up sweating from vivid nightmares, or their partner may complain that they walked, talked, or shouted—or even kicked or punched—during the night. Partners may say that these people seem to be acting out their dreams, especially scary ones. They sometimes discover that objects in their bedroom or in other rooms have moved or temporarily vanished, or they'll find half-eaten food or dirty dishes in the bedroom or kitchen. They may have vague memories of these events or no recollection whatso-ever. Such occurrences can be caused by what are known as para-somnias—a term broadly applied to range of unusual sleep-related events, most of which are covered in Chapter 14.

The parasomnias include those that occur during deep sleep (such as sleepwalking, sleep terrors, and confusional arousals); those that occur during REM sleep (REM sleep behavioral dis-order and nightmares); and other problems such as bruxism (grinding the teeth) and sleep-related eating disorders. These are the most common parasomnias:

- **Sleepwalking.** Sleepwalkers may carry out complex actions, such as moving furniture or leaving their residence, or they may simply pace back and forth by the bed.
- **Sleep terrors.** During these unsettling episodes, the sleeper typically sits up in bed and lets out a bloodcurdling scream. Sleep terrors may also be characterized by dilated pupils, rapid breathing, a racing heartbeat, sweating, and extreme confusion and agitation.
- **Confusional arousals.** Confusional arousals are events in which sleepers sit up in bed and act extremely disoriented. They don't respond to other people's voices and resist attempts at being comforted or consoled.
- **REM sleep behavior disorder.** Most people make subtle twitching movements during REM sleep. People with this disorder go further—shouting, punching, or otherwise acting out their dreams, putting themselves and their spouses at risk of injury.
- **Nightmares.** Nearly everyone has occasional nightmares, but they can be a problem if they are so frightening that the person dreads going to sleep or they occur so frequently that they cause sleep deprivation.
- **Sleep-related eating disorder.** This disorder prompts people to get out of bed while asleep and head for the refrigerator, where they often consume unhealthy, high-calorie food.

- **Bruxism.** This common condition can cause damage to teeth or the jaw, as well as make enough noise to wake up the sleeper's partner.
- **Other medical disorders (Chapter 19).** Health problems that raise an individual's risk of experiencing parasomnias include Parkinson's disease, Alzheimer's disease, and sleep fragmentation disorders such as sleep apnea. In addition, epilepsy can cause seizures during sleep.

I Can't Sleep Because of My Partner

People with sleep problems often disrupt their partner's sleep. Snoring and bruxism are the most common complaints, but people may also report getting kicked or punched or being roused from sleep by shouts or screams. Less dramatically, a severe insomniac's constant tossing and turning and frequent bathroom trips can impair a spouse's sleep.

When this is the primary complaint, it usually means the wrong person is in my office. If it's yours, give this book to your bed partner once you're finished.

By now you should have some leading suspects in your quest to learn which disorder lies at the root of your sleep difficulties. In the next chapter, we'll look at the most common sleep disorder of all—insomnia—and some possible treatments.

CHAPTER 8

Insomnia and Its Behavioral Treatments

"My sleep is so bad I can't function anymore."

"Nighttime is torture for me."

"If I don't get some sleep soon, I don't know what I am going to do."

"My health is falling to pieces because I can't sleep."

These are just some of the complaints I hear from people with insomnia. In this chapter, we'll look at insomnia and the non-pharmacologic treatments available to treat it. (We'll cover prescription sleep medications in Chapter 9 and alternative treatments in Chapter 10).

Defining and Classifying Insomnia

The word *insomnia* comes from the Latin *in* ("no") and *somnus* ("sleep") and literally it means "no sleep." Although people with insomnia often feel they get no sleep at all, most often the problem is difficulty getting enough restful sleep.

Everyone experiences a bad night or two of sleep now and then. These occasional bouts of insomnia can be caused by stress (such as the anticipation of starting a new job, the worry of los-

What Is Sunday Insomnia?

It is not unusual for people to have trouble falling asleep on Sunday nights. While anxiety about work or school on Monday is a potential cause, another important factor is often weekend changes in sleep habits. When someone stays up later Friday night and sleeps in Saturday morning, he or she is primed to stay up even later Saturday night and sleep in the next day. By Sunday evening, the body's clock is programmed to stay up late.

People who have developed a pattern of Sunday insomnia may feel their anxiety mount as they anticipate a difficult night ahead. The solution to the Sunday blues is to maintain your weekday rising schedule on the weekends. Then on Sunday night, if you have stayed on schedule, you should have no problem getting to sleep. If you have stayed up a bit later on Friday and Saturday, the sleep deprivation should help you get to sleep easily. In either case—and especially if getting anxious about the coming week interferes with getting to sleep—make sure to use the sleep hygiene/reconditioning tips described in this chapter to help avoid poor sleep.

ing the one you have, an impending marriage or house purchase, and so on); a new or disruptive sleep environment (such as trying to sleep in a hotel on a business trip); or disruption of your usual circadian cycle (such as jet lag after flying to Europe or problems caused by staying up late on weekends). When these occasional nights of poor sleep become regular occurrences, insomnia moves from a minor annoyance to a full-fledged sleep disorder.

Unlike many chronic health problems, such as asthma or diabetes, insomnia is not a single disorder or disease. Instead, it is a general symptom like fever or pain, with multiple potential causes. To qualify as insomnia, the situation must meet three requirements:

- You experience poor sleep, which can be difficulty falling or staying asleep, or poor-quality sleep in general.

- The problem occurs despite having an adequate opportunity and environment for sleep.
- The poor sleep results in some type of impairment while awake, such as fatigue, sleepiness, aches and pains, mood disturbances, poor concentration, impaired performance, lack of energy or motivation, or development of great concerns and worry about sleep.

If all three requirements are not met, there is probably another explanation for the problem. For instance, a person who complains that he feels fatigued and has no energy during the daytime but doesn't go to bed until 2 A.M. does not have insomnia; the self-induced chronic sleep deprivation is most likely responsible for the symptoms.

Insomnia can be classified by how long it lasts or by its source. In the case of duration, there are three categories:

- **Transient.** Lasting a few days
- **Short term.** Lasting a few weeks
- **Chronic.** Lasting more than three weeks

Transient insomnia usually accompanies some type of stress, like worrying about an upcoming test or an illness in the family. The problem should go away once the stress is relieved. The key is to maintain your regular schedule and avoid doing things that might compound the problem, such as doing chores late at night to make yourself sleepier or drinking caffeinated beverages in the late afternoon and evening to keep yourself awake.

With the longer lasting types of insomnia, the goal is to break the cycle of poor sleep that is starting to develop in short-term insomnia and is fully developed in chronic insomnia. In this cycle, poor sleep leads to feeling bad during the daytime, which in turn leads to worrying about whether or not you will sleep the next night. Often, bad habits develop that help perpetuate the cycle. Interventions can include behavioral treatments to correct bad sleep habits and reestablish your usual sleep/wake cycle or medications to interrupt the downward spiral.

Another, perhaps more helpful, way of classifying insomnia is by its source. Here, it broadly breaks into two categories: primary and secondary.

Primary Insomnia

Primary insomnia occurs independently and is not due to any other obvious cause. In rare cases, it begins in infancy, presumably because of an inborn abnormality of the mechanisms that control sleep. But in most cases, primary insomnia is "learned," meaning the condition develops over time during childhood or adulthood.

People who develop primary insomnia seem predisposed to the problem because they have overactive nervous systems. Studies of people with chronic insomnia show they have higher metabolic rates and produce higher levels of stress hormones than others. Some experience they've had triggers difficulty with sleep, though in most cases individuals can't recall a specific event. After experiencing a few sleepless nights, they learn to associate the bedroom with being awake. The usual cues to begin to relax, such as entering the bedroom, putting on pajamas or brushing their teeth, instead elicit anxiousness about whether or not sleep will come easily. This anxiety causes alertness rather than relaxation and can further interfere with sleep.

The same thing can occur upon waking during the night. Frequently checking the clock and watching time march by slowly is a constant reminder of not sleeping and brings on frustration and anxiousness about the lack of sleep. This alerting response makes it difficult, or even impossible, to fall back to sleep.

Misguided ways to cope with the sleep deprivation—such as drinking coffee, napping, going to bed earlier, having a nightcap, or staying in bed longer in the morning—only fuel the problem. As insomnia worsens, anxiety and frustration mount, leading to a vicious cycle in which fears about sleeplessness and its consequences perpetuate the insomnia.

Secondary Insomnia

Secondary insomnia results from another cause. Chronic second-ary insomnia is often caused by an illness or disease; it may be a sleep disorder (such as sleep apnea or narcolepsy), a nonsleep con-dition (such as angina, heartburn, or depression), or a medication taken for such a condition. Substances taken for reasons other than sleep or health—such as alcohol, caffeine, or recreational drugs—can also lead to the development of insomnia.

The most direct solution to secondary insomnia is to address the underlying source of sleeplessness. For example, if pain from arthritis keeps you awake, then treating the arthritis is the most effective way to improve your sleep. If a medication for depres-sion is keeping you awake, switching to a different medication that does not cause insomnia is advisable.

A report on insomnia issued after the 2005 National Institutes of Health State-of-the-Science Conference proposed using the term *comorbid insomnia* rather than secondary insomnia to describe sleep disturbances associated with other disorders. The proposal stems from several observations:

- The method by which other disorders cause insomnia isn't always clear.
- Insomnia often persists after resolution of the primary disorder.
- Considering insomnia to be a secondary disorder may lead to undertreatment of the insomnia because interventions focus mainly on the other disorder.

The important point to remember is that insomnia can develop along with other illnesses and should be addressed if treating the primary illness does not improve sleep.

Behavioral Treatments for Insomnia

Although there's a tendency to expect that medication will pro-vide the best solution to health problems, there are alternatives that work just as well (if not better) for chronic insomnia. Medications can be effective for short-term insomnia and have a role in trying to break the condition's downward cycle. However, the effectiveness of long-term use is not clear—it may even be harmful—and these medications can have significant side effects.

I strongly believe that behavioral treatments have significant advantages and should be explored early. Research has shown that behavioral treatments are as likely or more likely than medication to succeed over the long term, and they do not carry the health risks or side effects of sleeping pills. Although the behavioral treatments in this chapter are largely used to treat primary insomnia, they can also benefit people with secondary insomnia.

There is a host of behavioral treatments for insomnia. Some you can do on your own or with assistance from someone trained in behavioral therapy or stress reduction techniques; others require a psychologist or a sleep specialist trained in behavioral medicine (see Table 8.1).

TABLE 8.1 Behavioral Methods and Techniques and How You Learn Them

Method/Technique	How Best Provided
Sleep hygiene	Can be done alone, based on reading
	More effective with single instructional session from a primary care physician or sleep specialist
Progressive muscle relaxation Diaphragmatic breathing	Can be done alone, based on reading or audiotapes
Visualization	More effective with single instructional session with a sleep specialist or an instructor trained in stress reduction techniques
Reconditioning	Can be done alone, based on reading
Sleep restriction	More effective with multiple instructional sessions from a sleep specialist
Meditation	Can be done alone, based on reading or audiotapes
	More effective with single or multiple instructional sessions with a sleep specialist or an instructor trained in stress reduction techniques
Biofeedback	Requires multiple training sessions from a biofeedback specialist
Cognitive behavioral therapy	Requires multiple sessions (usually six or more) with a psychologist or sleep specialist trained in behavioral medicine

No single behavioral treatment has been shown to be significantly more effective than the others. Instead, all the treatments described in this section are liable to benefit some people who try them. The likelihood of a treatment's success largely depends on the individual's commitment to it, so you may have to do some trial and error to find the one that suits you best.

Sleep Hygiene

Insomnia can often be alleviated by maintaining good sleep hygiene. If you're not already familiar with these practices, I encourage you to review Chapter 6. In some cases, regular exercise, maintaining a regular sleep/wake routine, and avoiding sleep saboteurs are all you need to improve your ability to fall and stay asleep. In other cases, these tactics will need to be combined with other measures.

Reconditioning

In the 1970s, Northwestern University Professor Richard Bootzin developed a technique to train people with insomnia to break harmful associations between their sleep environment and wakefulness and frustration and to begin to associate the bedroom with sleep. Reconditioning, also known as "stimulus control," has six rules:

1. Go to bed only when you're sleepy.
2. Use the bed only for sleeping or sex. Do not read, watch television, eat, or worry in bed.
3. If you're unable to sleep quickly—within about twenty minutes—get up and move to another room. Stay up until you are sleepy, and then return to bed.
4. If you still can't fall asleep, repeat step 3 as often as necessary throughout the night.
5. During the reconditioning process, set your alarm and get up at the same time every morning, regardless of how much sleep you got during the night.
6. Do not nap during the day.

Case History

David, a twenty-four-year-old graduate engineering student at MIT, came to see me because he was having trouble going to sleep at night and getting up in the morning. He'd had this problem on and off for a decade, but it had gotten much worse over the last year. His sleep always worsened during stressful times, and he had found his last school year very taxing.

When David went to bed, his mind would start racing, thinking about the things he had to do the next day and how badly he needed to go to sleep. To compensate, he developed a routine of working on his computer in bed until 1 or 2 A.M. and then reading a book to try and make himself sleepy. After an hour and a half of reading, he would eventually fall asleep. (He had the light on a timer so he wouldn't have to get up to turn it off.) David would often wake up after a few hours and then be unable to get back to sleep. He'd then repeat the reading routine again.

David needed to get up for school by 8 or 9 A.M., but he always had trouble getting out of bed and would hit the snooze button repeatedly. Because he was only getting four or five hours of sleep each night, he was always tired. However, he had the same problem falling asleep even when he tried to nap.

Not surprisingly, David was having major academic problems. He was often late to class, fell behind in his assignments, and got

Each step builds on and reinforces the next, and all the steps must be followed for the technique to succeed. They establish a positive association between your bed and healthy sleep. By getting out of bed, the negative associations (frustration, irritation, and worrying about sleep) become associated with a site other than the bedroom. Be sure to do nonstimulating, relaxing things while you're awake to allow the sleep process to begin again. Maintaining a consistent sleep/wake routine and avoiding napping reestablishes a more normal pattern.

poor grades. At the time of our first meeting, he had taken a medical leave from school because he felt so lousy. David said he wasn't depressed and had no other medical problems—he was just worried about not sleeping.

It was clear that David had primary sleep onset and maintenance insomnia, and poor sleep hygiene and a delay in his circadian sleep phase were making the problem worse.

First we regularized his sleep routine and improved his sleep hygiene. I instructed him to work on the computer and read—and also to spend some time making notes on what he needed to remember the next day—*before* he got into bed. To improve his sleep efficiency, we also used some mild sleep restriction, limiting his time in bed to six hours. As his sleep improved, he increased his time in bed, making sure he still slept well at each new sleep duration.

When David returned six weeks later, he was much improved. It had taken a couple of weeks for things to get better, he said, but he was now going to bed at around 12:30, taking less than thirty minutes to fall asleep, and, if he awoke during the night, getting back to sleep without much difficulty. He was pleased with his progress and was planning to reenroll in school for the next semester.

Consistency is a key element to this technique's success. The six rules sound simple, but perfect compliance can be challenging. People are sometimes reluctant to get out of bed when they can't sleep. But those who are conscientious in following this regimen often find that reconditioning helps them return to a regular sleep schedule.

Sleep Restriction

People with insomnia tend to spend more time in bed, thinking they'll get enough sleep if they allow more time for it to happen.

This can be counterproductive and actually promote fragmented and poor-quality sleep.

Sleep restriction, which is based on the idea that spending less time in bed promotes more efficient sleep, takes the opposite approach. By curtailing the amount of time spent in bed, you learn to fall asleep quicker and sleep more soundly. As your sleep becomes more consolidated into a single block, the time in bed is slowly extended until you obtain a full night's sleep.

You start by estimating how much sleep you're getting. If it's five hours, and you need to wake up by 7 A.M., then on your first night of sleep restriction, you should go to bed at 2 A.M., no matter how sleepy you are before then. Once you sleep well during the allotted five hours for several days, you can add another fifteen or thirty minutes, making sure your sleep remains consolidated. Then repeat the process until you're up to the desired amount of sleep. If sleep grows fragmented again, take a step back until sleep becomes consolidated again.

If you're still having trouble falling or staying asleep at five hours, there may be something else going on, and you should check with your doctor. Spending less than five hours in bed is not recommended.

It's important not to sleep at other times, even though you may feel sleepy. You're using the homeostatic sleep drive to make you a more efficient nighttime sleeper—taking naps reduces this drive and can interfere with the technique's effectiveness.

Like reconditioning, sleep restriction seems simple in theory but can be challenging in practice, since people often have a hard time forcing themselves to stay awake for the first phase of the treatment. However, those who can stick with it often find it remarkably effective. Reconditioning and sleep restriction complement each other and are often prescribed simultaneously.

Relaxation Techniques
Insomnia that results from an anxious, stressed, or worried mind can often be addressed by learning ways to release physical ten-

sion, reduce arousal, and relax more effectively. Relaxation techniques should be done outside the bed and bedroom, prior to going to bed, to avoid actively "trying" to relax, which can interfere with sleep.

Methods include progressive muscle relaxation, deep breathing, meditation, visualization, and biofeedback. Use these techniques to reduce your level of arousal at bedtime.

Progressive Muscle Relaxation. This technique allows you to relax your entire body by tensing and relaxing a series of muscles. Follow these steps:

1. Find a place to sit or lie down and get into a comfortable position. Put a pillow under your head, or place one under your knees to relax your back. Rest your arms, with palms up, slightly apart from your body.
2. Take several slow, deep breaths through your nose. Exhale with a long sigh to release tension.
3. Begin to focus on your feet and ankles. Tighten the muscles briefly (five to ten seconds) and then relax them. Let them drop from your consciousness.
4. Slowly move your attention up through different parts of your body: your calves, thighs, lower back, hips, and pelvic area; your middle back, abdomen, upper back, shoulders, arms, and hands; your neck, jaw, tongue, forehead, and scalp.
5. If thoughts distract you, try to ignore them and return your attention to your breathing.

Deep Breathing. Also known as diaphragmatic breathing, this technique slows respiration, leading to relaxation and then sleep. The idea is to replicate the type of breathing you do when you're asleep (slow and predominantly from the diaphragm—the muscle between the abdomen and the chest), instead of the type you do when you're awake (faster and using the diaphragm and chest muscles). Follow these steps:

1. Start by finding a place where you can lie flat on your back with your feet slightly apart. Lightly rest one hand on your abdomen, just near your navel, and rest your other hand on your chest.
2. Inhale through your nose and calmly exhale through your mouth until you've emptied most of the air from your lungs. Focus on your breathing and watch which hand is moving. You want the hand on your chest to stay still or follow after the hand on your abdomen.
3. Gently inhale, slightly distending your abdomen to make it rise. Imagine warmth flowing into your lungs and all parts of your body. Pause for one second. Then, as you slowly count to four, gently exhale, letting your diaphragm relax and your abdomen slowly fall. Pause for another second.
4. Repeat this process five to ten times.

Meditation. There are many types of meditation that can reduce stress and help you relax just before bedtime. The specifics vary, but key steps typically include the following:

1. Sit somewhere quiet in comfortable, loose clothing.
2. Close your eyes, allow your hands to rest on your legs, and relax your muscles.
3. Take a deep breath and let it out slowly.
4. Choose a simple word such as *relax* or *easy*, a religious word or phrase, or a meaningless word like the mantra *om*. As you breathe, repeat the word aloud or in your mind.
5. Continue breathing regularly with your muscles relaxed. It may help to count your breaths, starting over with every five breaths.

Visualization. Also known as guided imagery, visualization is a form of meditation that helps you mentally remove yourself from stress. Follow these steps:

1. Sit or lie somewhere comfortable and close your eyes.
2. Imagine you are somewhere that makes you feel good, such as the beach or the woods, a spot where you have spent a restful vacation, or a beautiful place you can picture even if you have never been there.
3. Breathe slowly and deeply until you feel relaxed.
4. Focus on all five senses, imagining what you see, feel, hear, taste and smell. Continue to visualize yourself in this place for five to ten minutes.
5. Gradually return your focus to the room you are in.

Biofeedback. Most commonly used to treat migraine headaches, biofeedback is a form of therapy that teaches you to control physiological functions such as heart rate, muscle tension, breathing, perspiration, skin temperature, blood pressure, and even brain waves. By learning to control these functions, you may be able to reduce stress and improve sleep.

During biofeedback training, sensors placed on your body are attached to a machine to detect changes in your pulse, skin temperature, blood pressure, muscle activity, brain-wave pattern, or some other physiological function. These changes trigger a specific signal—a sound, a flashing light, or a change in pattern on a video screen—which tells you that the physiological change has occurred.

Gradually, with the help of your biofeedback therapist, you learn to alter the signal yourself by controlling your body's physiology. After a few sessions, there's no need for sensors or monitors, and you can use the same control techniques at home without supervision.

The success of the five relaxation methods presented here depends on whether you continue to practice them. It's common for people to begin with enthusiasm, achieve moderate success, but then fall back to their prior sleep level because they abandon the method or practice it much less frequently. These relaxation methods are not as effective as the behavioral methods described earlier, but people who continue to practice regularly are likely to be rewarded with improved sleep.

Cognitive Therapy

Cognitive therapy helps people learn new ways of thinking about and then doing things. It's been shown to be helpful in treating addictions, phobias, and anxiety—as well as insomnia.

Cognitive therapy for insomnia focuses on changing the negative thoughts and beliefs about sleep into positive ones. People with insomnia tend to become preoccupied with sleep and apprehensive about the consequences of poor sleep. This worry and apprehension heighten arousal and further hinder the ability to relax. Basic elements of cognitive therapy include setting realistic goals and learning to let go of inaccurate thoughts or beliefs that can interfere with sleep. Categories of some of the most common thoughts include:

- Misattributions, such as "When I feel anxious during the day, it's always because I did not sleep well the night before."
- Hopelessness, such as "I will never be able to get a decent night's rest tonight."
- Unrealistic expectations, such as "I have to get eight hours of sleep tonight" or "I have to fall asleep before my wife/husband does."
- Exaggerating consequences, such as "If I don't get to sleep soon, I'll embarrass myself at tomorrow's meeting."
- Performance anxiety, such as "It will take me at least an hour to fall asleep."

A cognitive behavior therapist helps you replace these maladaptive beliefs with accurate and constructive thoughts and habits, such as "All of my problems do not stem from insomnia," "I stand a good chance of getting a good night's sleep tonight," "My job does not depend on how much sleep I get tonight," and "Even if I don't fall asleep quickly tonight, it's not such a big deal." The therapist also provides structure and support while you practice the new thoughts and habits. Success requires practice and multiple sessions.

Cognitive therapy is often provided in combination with one or more behavioral therapies—what's known as cognitive behavioral therapy (CBT). Research has shown that CBT is more effective than any behavioral technique used by itself, and that it's more effective than sleeping pills. For example, a 2004 study of patients with insomnia who had five thirty-minute sessions over six weeks focusing on cognitive changes and reconditioning found that they were able to fall asleep in half the time it took before the study began, while patients who received a prescription medication cut that time by only 17 percent. CBT also led to improved sleep efficiency and fewer nighttime arousals.

The biggest obstacle to successful treatment with CBT is lack of patient commitment—some people fail to complete all the required sessions or to practice the techniques on their own. Those who do put forth the effort are likely to be rewarded.

As you saw in Table 8.1, you can learn many of these techniques on your own. After evaluating your sleep habits and making sure you have good sleep hygiene, you may wish to start out on your own or perhaps take a stress reduction class. Then, if you continue to have problems, speak to your doctor or a sleep specialist for more help.

CHAPTER 9

Medications for Treating Insomnia

Sleeping pills are among the most widely used drugs in the United States. About 10 percent of adults report using over-the-counter (OTC) sleep medications, and 10 percent use prescription medications. Usage appears to be increasing, especially among younger people. According to an independent group that monitors drug prescriptions, the number of adults age twenty to forty-four who use sleeping medications doubled from 2000 to 2004. Even though the total number is small, the number of children ages ten to nineteen who use sleeping pills rose by 85 percent during the same period.

If you have chronic insomnia, whether or not to take sleep medication is a decision you need to make in consultation with your doctor. It's not always an easy call. On the one hand, persistent sleeplessness can have negative physical and mental health effects and impair your quality of life, and sleeping pills can improve sleep. On the other hand, medications are not always effective and carry a number of drawbacks and health risks, so they're not an ideal solution for everyone.

My goal with this chapter is to give you an overview of the large and growing world of sleeping pills, so you can be an informed consumer in discussions with your physician. First, we'll

Menopause and Insomnia

Menopause is a time of major hormonal, physical, and psychological changes, and sleep disturbance is one of the hallmark symptoms. More than half of women complain of difficulty falling asleep, less restorative sleep, and daytime sleepiness during this life stage, and these sleep problems are frequently accompanied by depression and anxiety.

Sleep can also be disrupted by the most common manifestation of menopause—the hot flashes, hot flushes, and night sweats that occur in the majority of women. Hot flashes are unexpected feelings of heat all over the body. They are often accompanied by hot flushes: sweating and dilation of the blood vessels, which causes redness in the face, neck, and upper chest. These symptoms are caused by decreasing levels of estrogen.

Hormone replacement therapy (HRT) is the most frequent treatment for reducing menopausal symptoms, but its use is controversial. In addition to cutting a woman's risk of osteoporosis, HRT reduces the incidence of hot flashes, which improves sleep for some (but not all) women. However, research suggests that HRT

look at the key factors that distinguish sleeping pills in general. Then we'll go over the pros and cons of each class of medication. Finally, I'll show you what factors I take into account when deciding whether or not to prescribe sleep medication for my patients and what influences which drug I prescribe.

What Separates One Sleeping Pill from Another

Each class of sleep medication affects the body differently, and within the same class, there may be differences between specific drugs. Issues that distinguish sleeping pills include the following:

- **Effectiveness.** Along with the simple but important question of whether a medication makes you sleepy enough

may increase the risk of breast cancer, stroke, cardiovascular disease, and dementia.

If you take the lowest effective dose over the short term, you can reduce the health risks of HRT. If you're experiencing insomnia during menopause, discuss your options with your doctor, who can help you make informed decisions about use and dosage based on the severity of your symptoms and your family history of disease. No other medications are approved by the Food and Drug Administration (FDA) to treat hot flashes, but as an alternative to HRT, your doctor may recommend medications that decrease their intensity, such as clonidine, gabapentin, or antidepressants. The sleeping medications described in this chapter may also be used to improve sleep in the menopausal period, but they do not affect the other menopausal symptoms.

One final note: The incidence of sleep apnea in women increases significantly after menopause. Be on the lookout for the signs of this disorder (see Chapter 11) so you can get proper treatment if needed.

to nod off is the more complex issue of how it works in terms of onset and duration. Some pills take effect within ten minutes, while others take an hour or more. Some wear off quickly (in one to five hours), while others last much longer (six to eight hours or more). A medication's half-life—how long it takes for half the drug to leave your body—can help patients evaluate its duration. The effect should suit an individual's sleep problem, with fast-acting drugs benefiting people who have trouble falling asleep and longer lasting pills aiding those who have difficulty staying asleep.

- **Impact on sleep quality.** On the plus side, sleeping pills reduce the time it takes to fall asleep and the number of nighttime arousals, and they can extend sleep time. On the minus side, they change sleep architecture. Most commonly, they increase the amount of time you spend in Stage 1 and 2 sleep and decrease the time spent in deep sleep and REM sleep. As long as the benefit of increased total sleep outweighs the drawback of decreased deep sleep, you'll be better off. In practice, it depends on your particular sleep problem and how you respond to the medication.

- **Tolerance.** With some sleep medication, the drug becomes less effective over time and you need more and more of it to obtain the same effect. This phenomenon is known as tolerance, and it happens commonly with drugs that affect the central nervous system. Physical changes occur that make the brain less sensitive to the drug. When this takes place, a higher dose is needed to trigger the same response. Depending on the individual and the medication, tolerance can take anywhere from a week or two to several months to develop. In some cases, even higher doses no longer have any effect.

- **Rebound.** Stopping sleep medication abruptly after long-term use can cause some people to experience insomnia that's even worse than the insomnia they had before they started the regimen. This rebound insomnia, which usually lasts only a few days, may be accompanied by muscle tension, restlessness, irritability, or, in rare cases, convulsions. Slowly tapering down the amount of the medicine allows people to avoid this reaction.

- **Dependence.** People sometimes become convinced that they can't possibly get a good night's sleep without pharmaceutical assistance. Such a strong reluctance to stop use is referred to as dependence, and it can trap people in a vicious cycle. If they stop the medication for a night, they experience rebound insomnia and sleep poorly. The next day they feel so tired that they restart the medication to get a good night's sleep. The poor sleep without medication reinforces the belief that they can't sleep without it. The likelihood of dependence varies with the different classes of drugs. Although powerful, the dependence prompted by sleeping pills is psychological, unlike the physical addiction that can develop with nicotine or heroin.

- **Safety.** The sedation caused by sleeping pills can reduce reaction time and coordination and impair judgment while the drug is on board, leading to problems driving, operating machinery, and making decisions. To avoid these risks, it's important to set aside enough time to get adequate sleep and to allow the medication to wear off. Several studies have suggested that sleeping pills may increase the risk of falls in the elderly, a population already at high risk for falls, and two large population studies found an association between the use of sleeping pills and higher death rates (although it wasn't clear whether sleeping pills caused higher death rates or were simply more likely to be used by very ill people). Such research shouldn't dissuade you from using medication, but it serves as a reminder to use it appropriately and in consultation with your doctor.

- **Side effects.** Like all medications, sleeping pills can cause unwanted side effects. The most common is grogginess upon waking—also known as "morning hangover"—which results from the medication lingering in your body beyond your preferred wake-up time. Other frequent side effects include dizziness, dry mouth, and upset stomach. Lastly, the active ingredients in sleeping pills can counteract or enhance the effects of other medications (and alcohol), so it's important to inform your doctor about any other prescription or OTC medications —including allergy medicine, diet pills, and so on—you use before you start taking a sleeping pill.

Over-the-Counter Medications

Despite the large number of competing brands of OTC sleep medications, this class of products is surprisingly straightforward. Each one—whether it's a tablet, capsule, or gelcap—contains an antihistamine as its primary active ingredient (see Table 9.1). Most OTC sleep aids (including Nytol, Sominex, and numerous generic versions) contain the antihistamine diphenhydramine. A few, such as Unisom SleepTabs, contain doxylamine, another antihistamine. Others (including Aspirin-Free Anacin PM and Extra Strength Tylenol PM) combine the same antihistamines with the pain reliever acetaminophen.

Antihistamines are widely used to treat allergies in drugs such as Benadryl and its generic equivalents. They block the release of histamine, a chemical produced by the body in reaction to foreign substances known as allergens, reducing swelling of the nasal passages and making it easier to breathe. But antihistamines have a side effect—they also block the wake-enhancing effect of histamine in the sleep regulating centers, causing drowsiness. For insomniacs, this incidental effect of allergy treatment becomes the prime reason to take the medication.

While OTC antihistamines are reasonably effective in helping people fall and stay asleep after a single administration, little research has been done on their long-term effectiveness or safety. They can cause all the drawbacks listed earlier: morning hangover, tolerance, and dependence. Tolerance to the sleepiness side effect develops quickly, on average in about four days. These drugs have

TABLE 9.1 Over-the-Counter Sleep Medications

Brand	Active Ingredient	Onset of Action (minutes)	Half-Life (hours)	Side Effects
Nytol QuickCaps	Diphenhydramine	15–30	3–12	Common: nausea, dizziness, gastric distress, dry mouth, disturbed coordination
Simply Sleep				
Sleepinal Maximum Strength Softgels				
Sominex Maximum Strength Caplets				Rare: fast or irregular heartbeat, blurred vision, delirium, sensitivity to sunlight
Tylenol PM				
Unisom SleepGels, Maximum Strength				
Unisom SleepTabs	Doxylamine			

a high rate of side effects, including nausea, dizziness, gastric distress, dry mouth, and disturbed coordination.

So while there's no great danger in using an antihistamine for a night or two to treat an occasional bout of insomnia, I advise against using them any more often than that. If you do ultimately choose to take medication to combat chronic insomnia, prescription drugs are preferable because they have been shown to be effective and carry fewer drawbacks.

Prescription Medications

Prescription medications for insomnia break down into four general classes: benzodiazepine receptor agonists, antidepressants, melatonin receptor agonists, and barbiturates.

Benzodiazepine Receptor Agonists

Agonists are drugs that bind to a receptor site on a cell and cause an action to occur. Benzodiazepine receptor agonists work by increasing the efficiency of gamma-aminobutryric acid (GABA), a neurotransmitter that reduces how often neurons fire alertness-promoting messages to each other. The drugs attach themselves to receptor sites on nerve cell molecules, changing the shape of the site slightly, so it's more attractive to GABA molecules. The binding of GABA opens pores in the cell, allowing chloride ions to flow into the cell, which makes the cell less likely to react. Depending on the cell's location, GABA binding can lead to sedation, muscle relaxation, decreased anxiety, and antiseizure effects.

Until recently, benzodiazepines—which have been available since the 1960s—were the only prescription drugs specifically approved for insomnia. This class of medications is proven effective in making people fall asleep faster, wake up less often, and sleep longer overall. There are two types: benzodiazepine hypnotics and nonbenzodiazepine hypnotics. While nonbenzodiazepines have a different structure and therefore are not technically benzodiazepines, their action on cells is so similar that most physicians put them in the same general class.

Case History

Donna was an emergency room doctor whose sleep problem began shortly after the birth of her son. Before that, she'd always been a good sleeper. But after getting up during the night for several months to feed her baby, Donna was unable to return to a normal routine once her son started sleeping through the night. She would wake up on her own several times a night and then have trouble getting back to sleep.

The problem steadily worsened. When Donna got into bed, she would lie awake going over her to-do list. She watched the clock march the night away and grew frustrated at not sleeping well. She got jealous of how easily her husband fell asleep next to her, making it even harder to get to sleep, and her tossing and turning disturbed his sleep. This nightly sleep battle created friction between the couple, prompting her to move to another room so that he could sleep.

Donna's work schedule made the problem worse. Twice a week, she worked a shift from 2 P.M. to 2 A.M. On these late nights, it took her a while to wind down and more than an hour to fall asleep. The schedule and the poor sleep took their toll—she felt tired a lot and always had a hard time getting up.

Donna's physician diagnosed her with chronic sleep onset insomnia. He observed that her sleep was initially disrupted by the stress of caring for her baby, but then she became conditioned to sleep poorly. The doctor gave her a trial of Ambien for two weeks and she slept very well. However, the problem recurred once she stopped taking it. He then switched her to longer-lasting Lunesta;

Benzodiazepine Hypnotics. Currently nine benzodiazepine medications are available (see Table 9.2 on page 104). Five are FDA approved to treat short-term insomnia: estazolam (ProSom), flurazepam (Dalmane), quazepam (Doral), temazepam (Restoril), and triazolam (Halcion). Four others are approved to treat anxiety: clonazepam (Klonopin), lorazepam (Ativan), alprazolam (Xanax),

she fell asleep quickly and slept through the night but woke up feeling groggy. She tried to wean herself off Lunesta, but she woke up during the night with lower doses and slept poorly again when she didn't take anything.

By this point, Donna was exhausted physically and emotionally. Her doctor referred her to me, hoping a different approach might yield better results.

After my evaluation, Donna and I agreed to try combining pharmacologic and behavioral treatments. She switched back to the short-acting Ambien to avoid the morning grogginess, and she only used the medication after her late shift and the following night to guarantee sleep on her toughest nights. On other nights, she restricted her time in bed to six hours, the amount she had been sleeping, to consolidate her sleep into a single block. We also worked to change her association of bed as a place of frustration by having her not stay in bed if she couldn't sleep.

Although skeptical, Donna followed the regimen faithfully. In about two weeks, she noticed that she was sleeping through the night without medication and getting to sleep quicker. She slowly extended her sleep time. When I saw her a month later, she was using the medication only to help with shift work. The other nights she was regularly falling asleep in less than fifteen minutes and awaking refreshed seven and a half to eight hours later. Pleased with her progress, she left my office ready to move back into her bedroom with her husband.

and diazepam (Valium). Because doctors are free to prescribe approved drugs however they see fit—which is called off-label use —these four are also sometimes prescribed for patients who have trouble sleeping.

Benzodiazepines differ in how quickly they kick in and how long they remain active in the body. For example, Halcion is

TABLE 9.2 Benzodiazepine Hypnotics

Generic Name	Brand Name	Onset of Action (minutes)	Half-Life (hours)	Side Effects
Alprazolam	Xanax	60–120	11–20	Clumsiness or unsteadiness, dizziness, light-headedness, daytime drowsiness, headache
Clonazepam	Klonopin	30–60	30–40	
Diazepam	Valium	30–60	30–100	
Estazolam*	ProSom	15–30	8–24	
Flurazepam*	Dalmane	15–45	48–120	
Lorazepam	Ativan	15–45	8–12	
Quazepam*	Doral	15–30	48–120	
Temazepam*	Restoril	45–50	8–20	
Triazolam*	Halcion	15–30	2–6	

*FDA approved for the treatment of insomnia.

absorbed into the bloodstream in about ten minutes and has a short half-life (about five hours), so it begins working quickly and is short-acting. As a result, it's often used to treat people who have trouble falling asleep. By contrast, Restoril has a slower absorption rate and a half-life of about eight hours, so it's often used to treat people who have trouble staying asleep. Drugs with very long half-lifes, like Dalmane and Doral, are more likely to cause morning grogginess and daytime sleepiness.

In the short term, benzodiazepines are usually effective in helping people fall and stay asleep. Since they reduce anxiety, they tend to be especially useful for patients whose insomnia stems from this disorder.

However, they carry many of the same drawbacks as antihistamines: a reduction in the amount of deep sleep, a potential for morning hangover (which sometimes continues all day long), and rebound. These drawbacks take longer to develop than they do with antihistamines but can be more severe. Although tolerance has long been a concern with benzodiazepines, most studies do not show escalation in the amount of medicine people take. However, it's clear that some people do develop dependence with long-term use and have difficulty discontinuing use.

Reported side effects include unsteadiness, dizziness, amnesia for events occurring after taking a dose, light-headedness, and headaches. Benzodiazepines are safe unless mixed with alcohol. This combination can be dangerous—even fatal. People with untreated sleep apnea should not use them because of their muscle relaxant effect, and people with other breathing difficulties should use caution because of their mild respiratory depressant effect. Finally, bear in mind that all of these medications are only approved for short-term use; their effectiveness beyond a couple of weeks has rarely been tested.

Nonbenzodiazepine Hypnotics. These medications come from a relatively new class of drugs that resemble benzodiazepines in their ability to enhance the sleep-inducing activity of the neurotransmitter GABA but have a slightly different chemical composition. While benzodiazepines have a generalized effect on multiple brain receptors, the nonbenzodiazepines act only on the specific receptors in your brain that focus on sleep, leading to fewer side effects. They also appear to have little or no effect on deep sleep.

Many physicians now prescribe nonbenzodiazepine hypnotics in situations where they formerly prescribed benzodiazepines. Currently, three are available (see Table 9.3). Zolpidem (Ambien) was the first to gain FDA approval in 1992, followed by zaleplon (Sonata) in 1999 and eszopiclone (Lunesta) in 2004. Additional drugs in this class are likely to be released in coming years.

Sonata and Ambien both act quickly (within twenty minutes) and largely wear off before the end of a usual night of sleep. Sonata wears off especially quickly—for this reason, it won't keep you asleep for the whole night if you take it before you go to bed,

TABLE 9.3 Nonbenzodiazepine Hypnotics*

Generic Name	Brand Name	Onset of Action (minutes)	Half-Life (hours)	Side Effects
Eszopiclone	Lunesta	30	5–7	Headache,
Zaleplon	Sonata	10–20	1	daytime drowsiness,
Zolpidem	Ambien	10–20	1.5–2.4	dizziness, nausea
	Ambien CR	10–20	3	

*All are FDA approved for the treatment of insomnia.

Ambien and Sleep Eating

Several news reports in 2006 drew attention to an unusual side effect of Ambien use, sleep eating. In these cases, people were witnessed foraging for food at night but were unable to remember the episodes in the morning or they reported finding evidence of a midnight feast in the kitchen without any recollection of participating in it. Several people reported significant weight gains.

Sleep eating is a parasomnia—a sleep disorder that causes people to do unusual things during partial arousal from sleep without memory of the behavior the next morning (see Chapter 14). The link between Ambien and sleep eating actually dates to 2002, when doctors at the Mayo Clinic reported the phenomenon in five patients with restless leg syndrome who had begun taking the medication. The sleep eating ceased when they stopped using Ambien.

Since then, other investigators have reported similar cases of sleep eating. Additional unusual side effects seen with Ambien (as well as other benzodiazepine receptor agonists) include sleep walking, short-term amnesia, and, rarely, sleep driving. Some of the driving cases occurred when people took sleep medication after drinking alcohol.

Overall, the number of these cases is small given the millions of prescriptions written yearly for Ambien. Though rare, they highlight the need for people who use sleep medication to use it properly and be aware of potential side effects. Always allow enough time for sleep, use only as directed, and avoid alcohol. If you experience any unusual occurrences, talk to your doctor right away.

but you can take one if you wake up in the middle of the night and can't go back to sleep. Lunesta takes a little longer to kick in and also lasts longer. A long-acting version of Ambien (Ambien CR) became available in 2005 to treat problems with sleep maintenance as well as sleep onset insomnia. While all three medications make you fall asleep more quickly, only Ambien CR and Lunesta increase total sleep time.

Another difference is that while Ambien and Sonata are both approved to treat only short-term insomnia, Lunesta is approved to treat insomnia for up to six months. This does not mean Lunesta is necessarily superior—just that its manufacturer took the time and expense to conduct studies demonstrating that it's safe and effective for longer use.

While nonbenzodiazepines carry fewer drawbacks than anti-histamines or benzodiazepines, they're not perfect for everyone. Some people find they're not powerful enough to induce sleep. Even with the shorter half-life, some people may still experience morning grogginess, tolerance, and rebound, as well as side effects such as headache, dizziness, and nausea. Another issue is that since the nonbenzodiazepines are relatively new, we don't know their long-term effects. Even so, they have quickly become the most commonly prescribed benzodiazepine receptor agonist medications.

Antidepressants

Physicians increasingly prescribe antidepressant medications to patients with insomnia, usually at a lower dose than would typically be used to treat depression. While benzodiazepines were the most commonly prescribed sleep medications in the 1980s, doctors changed their patterns during the 1990s, and by 2002, three of the top five most frequently prescribed sleep medications were antide-pressants. This occurred even though antidepressants are neither FDA approved for nor proven effective for treating insomnia.

Several factors influenced this trend. Some doctors have the perception that antidepressants have fewer side effects and are safer for long-term use than benzodiazepines and that all insomnia is related to depression. None of these beliefs is supported by con-vincing evidence. Another factor is that there are fewer regula-tory restrictions for antidepressants than for benzodiazepines, so they're easier to prescribe.

Despite the lack of research on their effectiveness against insomnia, antidepressants do seem to help some people. Studies of depressed people who also have sleep problems show that the medication reduces sleep latency and nighttime arousals. How they cause sleepiness isn't clear, but it may be due to a sedative effect. It may also result from the drugs' easing of anxiety and mild depression, which makes it easier for sleepers with these problems to relax and fall asleep.

Antidepressants' effect on sleep quality varies—in general, they reduce REM sleep but have minimal impact on deep sleep. They often cause side effects, the most common of which are dizziness, dry mouth, upset stomach, weight gain, and sexual dysfunction (see Table 9.4). They also can increase leg movements

TABLE 9.4 Antidepressants Used to Treat Insomnia*

Type	Generic Name	Brand Name	Most Common Side Effects
Serotonin modulator	Trazodone	Desyrel	Dizziness, dry mouth, headache, nausea, constipation or diarrhea, painful erections
Selective serotonin reuptake inhibitor (SSRI)	Fluoxetine	Prozac	Dry mouth, drowsiness, dizziness, sexual dysfunction, nausea, diarrhea, headache, jitteriness, sweating, insomnia, weight gain
	Sertraline	Zoloft	
	Fluvoxamine	Luvox	
	Paroxetine	Paxil	
	Citalopram	Celexa	
Serotonin and norepinephrine reuptake inhibitor (SNRI)	Venlafaxine	Effexor	Upset stomach, excitement or anxiety, nightmares, dry mouth, skin sensitivity to sunlight, weight gain, headache
Tetracyclic	Mirtazapine	Remeron	Dry mouth, constipation, weight gain, headache, dizziness
Tricyclic	Amitriptyline	Elavil, Endep	Dry mouth, dizziness, constipation, incomplete urination, weight gain, sun sensitivity, sweating, faintness on standing, increased heart rate, sexual dysfunction
	Doxepin	Sinequan	
	Nortriptyline	Pamelor	
	Trimipramine	Surmontil	

*Not FDA approved to treat insomnia but often prescribed for patients with this condition.

during sleep. Some people find certain antidepressants make them feel nervous or restless, so the medication can actually exacerbate insomnia. It's not clear whether these medications lead to tolerance or rebound insomnia.

Melatonin Receptor Agonist

The new drug Rozerem (ramelteon) is the first drug in a class known as melatonin receptor agonists, the first new sleep medication class in thirty years. Rozerem is approved to treat insomnia for people who have trouble falling asleep at bedtime (sleep onset insomnia).

Rozerem works by attaching to the same receptors on the suprachiasmatic nucleus as the body's naturally produced melatonin does. The SCN is the site in the brain that controls the circadian cycle of sleep and wakefulness (see Chapter 2). Rozerem has a more potent effect on the SCN than ingested melatonin, which reduces sleep latency in some people and can be used to change the circadian sleep phase.

Because Rozerem doesn't act on the benzodiazepine receptor or involve GABA, its side effect profile is different. The most common side effect is dizziness, and there is a risk that it may exacerbate symptoms of depression. Also, people with severe liver damage or those who are using the antidepressant fluvoxamine (Luvox) shouldn't take it. Rozerem has a short half-life of two to five hours. Citing clinical studies that found that Rozerem did not cause tolerance, dependence, or rebound insomnia, the drug's manufacturer promotes it for long-term use.

Researchers have yet to compare Rozerem to other sleep medications, so too little information is available to determine the drug's role in the pharmacologic treatment of insomnia. It may be more likely to benefit older people than younger people, since people produce less melatonin as they age. However, older people's primary sleep problem tends to be waking up during the night (not falling asleep at bedtime), suggesting that Rozerem's usefulness may be limited. More studies and clinical experience should help clarify the picture.

TABLE 9.5 Barbiturates

Generic Name	Brand Name	Side Effects
Pentobarbital	Nembutal	Common: unsteadiness, dizziness, light-
Phenobarbital	Barbita, Luminal, Solfoton	headedness, grogginess, anxiety, constipation, headache, irritability, nausea
		Also: Habit forming; can be fatal if taken in combination with alcohol; possible
Secobarbital	Seconal	delirium or convulsions from abrupt discontinuation

Barbiturates

Drugs in this class (see Table 9.5) have been available for nearly a century and were a common ingredient in sleep medications until benzodiazepines reached the market. Barbiturates carry numerous drawbacks, including reduced sleep quality, morning hangover, and tolerance. More importantly, barbiturates are highly addictive, discontinuing use can be painful and difficult, and an overdose is often fatal. Today, sleep experts rarely prescribe barbiturates.

On the Horizon

Many new sleep agents are in the pipeline and should be available in the next few years. Companies continue to develop new benzodiazepine receptor agonists to improve the specificity of the drugs and reduce side effects. We should see a new drug called gaboxadol that stimulates GABA activity at an entirely new receptor site. Drugs used to treat other health problems also may have benefits for insomniacs. And as our understanding of the brain and sleep continues to improve, new sites of action will be identified that may be susceptible to medication.

My Perspective on Sleep Medication

While there's no doubt that insomnia is a significant problem, I'm concerned that the current onslaught of television and magazine ads telling people to ask their doctors for sleeping pills gives the false impression that a pill is all that's needed. Physicians often prescribe these medications without doing a thorough evaluation of the complaint. I'm not opposed to patients using sleeping pills, but I do want to make sure they get the right treatment. Accordingly, I always consider several key questions before prescribing sleep medication:

- **What is the source of insomnia?** One of the first things I discuss with patients is what effort was made to determine the insomnia's source. If the insomnia is a result of another treatable illness or a side effect of a medication for such an illness—that is, it's a case of secondary insomnia—then we need to focus on addressing the primary source. In many cases, doing so will resolve the insomnia without the need for sleeping pills.
- **What other treatments have been tried?** By the time people get to my office, they have usually been suffering from insomnia for a long time. As a result, most have experimented with many over-the-counter treatments, tried lots of home remedies, and received multiple courses of sleep medications from their primary care physicians. Often, they've been on sleep medications for so long that they have difficulty stopping use, and reliance on sleeping pills has become part of the problem.

  After reviewing what's been tried, it's important to identify what has worked and what hasn't. People who experience significant rebound when trying to stop medication need to taper off the medication slowly. Sometimes changing the dosage of a current prescription can help, but in general, medications that haven't worked in the past are unlikely to work in the future no matter what strength or amount is given. Recognition of side effects can also help identify appropriate agents.

  I also always ask patients who request sleeping pills if they're practicing good sleep hygiene (see Chapter 6) and what, if any, behavioral treatments (see Chapter 8) they've tried. If these areas haven't been explored, medication may not be needed.

- **What are the patient's treatment goals?** It's important to set realistic goals or you'll inevitably be disappointed and consider worthwhile improvements a failure. Too often, people's expectations—such as falling asleep as soon as they get into bed, always getting eight hours of sleep, or never waking up during the night—are unrealistic. The goal should be to get enough good-quality sleep to feel rested during the daytime. Sleep medication is just one tool to achieve this goal.

Selecting the Right Medication

If I decide that sleep medication is warranted, here's how the different classes of drugs typically come in to play. Benzodiazepine receptor agonists are the first medications considered for insomnia. For problems with sleep onset only, I will choose one of the short-acting agents, such as Halcion, Sonata, or Ambien. For problems staying asleep or early-morning awakenings, I select a medium-acting agent such as Restoril or Lunesta.

Antidepressants are the second medications to consider. I prescribe these if benzodiazepines don't work or have unacceptable side effects. In addition, I sometimes use antidepressants in special situations, such as for people who have respiratory disease or untreated sleep apnea, a history of substance abuse, or a coexisting emotional problem.

The role of the melatonin receptor agonist is not yet clear, but it will likely be used in the treatment of people with sleep onset insomnia.

On rare occasions, insomnia may be so severe that it requires combination therapy with multiple medications, such as a benzodiazepine and an antidepressant. In such cases, I usually encourage the individual to try cognitive behavioral therapy as well.

Dosing Instructions

Once the appropriate medication is determined, I give patients the following advice:

- **Don't exceed the dosage.** Physicians prescribe the lowest effective dose, so taking more without consulting your doctor can raise safety issues.
- **Use at bedtime.** Unless otherwise instructed, don't wait until you're in bed and having trouble falling asleep to decide whether to take the medication. This can perpetuate concern about sleep, delay the onset of action, and make morning grogginess more likely.
- **Take a short-term approach.** Use the medication until the problem resolves, up to about two to four weeks. Within that time frame, the likelihood of rebound or tolerance is small.
- **Consult a doctor about further use.** Improvement of sleep with short-term use, coupled with addressing sleep disturbance issues and improving sleep behaviors, is usually sufficient. However, after initial correction of the problem, intermittent use might be required if the insomnia returns.

Although I usually advise against continued long-term use, this is beneficial in rare cases, such as when behavioral treatments and trials of withdrawing medications have both been unsuccessful. Insomniacs who require long-term use should have ongoing monitoring by their physician or a sleep specialist. Be sure to consult with your doctor about the pros and cons of both intermittent and long-term use.

CHAPTER 10

Alternative Insomnia Treatments

People have used plants, herbs, and other methods to try to heal or cure themselves for thousands of years. It's not surprising that they're willing to try alternative treatments for insomnia as well. If you're considering an alternative therapy, you're probably wondering, "Can they help me sleep?"

This is a difficult question to answer. Unfortunately, few rigorous studies have examined whether alternative therapies actually benefit people with insomnia (or other chronic health problems, for that matter). Alternative therapies are not strictly regulated by the federal government, so practitioners and manufacturers have little incentive to conduct large and costly studies to prove that their techniques and products are safe and effective. Without solid research, we're largely left with anecdotal evidence, which makes it hard for physicians to make fact-based judgments.

When patients ask me about trying an alternative therapy, I urge them to keep three things in mind:

- Make sure the treatment is not potentially dangerous. Most are not, but occasionally reports of problems surface, such as those that led the FDA to warn against using supplements containing kava in 2002. The herb, used for relaxation and stress reduction, was linked to twenty-five cases of liver damage.

- Use alternative therapies in conjunction with conventional treatments, not in place of them. If you've recently improved your sleep hygiene, don't revert to bad habits because you're trying acupuncture.

- Always let your doctor know if you're using an alternative therapy, in case it's known to interact with any medication you're taking. For example, some herbs can decrease the anticlotting effect of the drug warfarin (Coumadin), increasing the risk of a blood clot.

A rundown of the alternative treatments most often used by people with insomnia follows.

Herbal Supplements

Herbal supplements are the leading form of alternative health therapy, and their use drives a multibillion-dollar industry. Even so, FDA regulation of herbs remains limited. According to the 1994 Dietary Supplement Health and Education Act, manufacturers do not have to prove that the supplement works. As long as the product label doesn't make unsupported scientific claims, manufacturers have a great deal of leeway in promoting their products' alleged benefits. The FDA must prove an herb unsafe to remove it from the market.

So consumers need to exercise care when making a purchase. Because supplements' ingredients and purity can vary greatly among manufacturers, it's best to buy products that say "standardized extracts" on the label. Note that a supplement's effectiveness may vary from brand to brand, even if the dosage is the same.

The case of L-tryptophan, a supplement promoted as a safe and natural sleep agent in the late 1980s, illustrates this point. The body breaks down this chemical to make serotonin, a neurotransmitter that promotes sleepiness. In 1989, hundreds of patients who had taken L-tryptophan required hospitalization for a strange group of symptoms that included intense muscle and joint pain, skin rash, swelling of the face and extremities, and shortness of breath due to fluid in the lungs. Blood tests showed high levels of eosinophils, blood cells that often increase during allergic reactions. Although the exact cause of the reaction to L-tryptophan was never proven conclusively, investigators suspect contaminants introduced during the manufacturing process played a role. Once the supplement was removed from the market, no further cases occurred. However, thirty-eight people died and a large number of those who survived were left with permanent disabilities.

If you take herbs to ease insomnia or with other goals in mind (increased energy, enhanced memory, and so on), I want to emphasize the importance of keeping your doctor informed. As noted earlier, herbs can interact with medications you may be taking. It's unwise to combine them with prescription sleep medications, since you may end up with an overly powerful sedative effect that makes it hard to get up in the morning. Herbs also can affect preexisting health conditions, including hypertension and diabetes. They can increase bleeding during surgery, so it's crucial that your physician know what you're taking if you're planning to have an operation. Finally, women who are pregnant, nursing, or trying to get pregnant should be especially wary of herbs' potential dangers and discuss any use with their obstetrician.

The herbs most frequently claimed to alleviate insomnia are valerian, lavender, chamomile, and passionflower.

- **Valerian.** A perennial plant native to Europe and Asia that has an unpleasant odor, valerian's use as a medicinal herb dates at least as far back as ancient Greece and Rome; in the second century, the Greek physician and philosopher Galen prescribed it for insomnia. Today, preparations from its roots and stems are put into capsules and tablets or are used to make tea.

  A few small studies suggest valerian is mildly sedating and can help people fall asleep and improve their sleep quality.

However, a 2005 review in the *Journal of Clinical Sleep Medicine* pointed out that most of the studies were small and flawed and that even the positive studies showed only a mild effect. The review also noted that valerian contains dozens of substances, and there's no scientific agreement on which of its constituents affect the human body. Also, the National Institutes of Health's (NIH's) 2005 State-of-the-Science Conference statement on insomnia notes that "limited evidence [on valerian] shows no benefit compared with placebo." The most commonly reported side effects are headaches, dizziness, itching, and gastrointestinal disturbances.

As with other unregulated remedies, the quality of valerian-containing products varies widely. A report by ConsumerLab—a commercial laboratory that periodically tests the quality of herbal remedies—found that nearly a quarter of valerian-based products appeared to contain no valerian whatsoever, and an equal number had less than half the amount claimed on their labels.

- **Lavender.** This shrub flourishes throughout southern Europe, Australia, and the United States. Its pleasant aroma, which comes from the oil in its small, blue-violet flowers, is often used in soaps, bath gels, and shampoos. Lavender is used in several ways by people with insomnia. Some use the flowers to make tea. Others put several drops of oil in boiling water and inhale the vapors or apply the oil directly to the skin during a massage. Whichever method is used, proponents claim lavender makes them feel relaxed, leading to restful sleep. Side effects are rare but can include nausea, headache, and chills.

- **Chamomile.** A daisylike plant that grows in Europe, chamomile has been used for thousands of years to treat everything from digestive disorders to skin conditions to insomnia. Most commonly its dried flowers are used to make tea, which purportedly helps bring on drowsiness. While generally considered safe, highly concentrated chamomile tea may cause vomiting. Also, people who are allergic to ragweed should avoid it because it's in the same plant family and may prompt an allergic reaction.

- **Passionflower.** A perennial climbing vine with a wood stem that grows to nearly thirty feet, passionflower grows in Europe and in the southeastern regions of North America. Preparations made from its flowers, leaves, and stems can be used to make tea or taken in a capsule. Passionflower is mainly used to treat insomnia and anxiety (often in combination with valerian). Side effects are rare but include nausea and rapid heartbeat.

I often hear from patients that they would prefer a "natural" cure. Bear in mind that all supplements work by providing some type of chemical. To my mind, a chemical that comes from a plant is no more natural—nor any safer or more likely to work—than one synthesized in a lab. What matters is whether what you're taking into your body has been demonstrated to be safe and effective. In truth, the most natural cure is to change your behavior to reestablish a regular schedule and good sleep habits.

In summary, with the exception of a possible mild benefit from valerian, very little scientific data backs the use of herbal treatments for insomnia, and some of them have significant potential adverse side effects. For more information about the safety and effectiveness of herbal therapies, I recommend looking at the websites of the NIH's Office of Dietary Supplements (ods.od.nih.gov), the American Herbal Products Association (ahpa.org), and ConsumerLab (consumerlab.com).

Synthetic Melatonin

As you'll recall from Chapter 2, melatonin is a hormone secreted by the pineal gland in the brain. Production peaks in the late evening, in conjunction with the onset of sleep. Since the 1990s, a synthetic version has been widely available in the United States as a supplement at health food stores and pharmacies. As a food supplement, there is no regulation of the amount or quality of the melatonin in each tablet. In Great Britain and Canada, melatonin is classified as a medicine and available by prescription only.

Although some researchers initially expressed enthusiasm for synthetic melatonin's possible role as an insomnia treatment, most subsequent research has been disappointing, finding either minimal benefits or none at all. A 2004 review of the melatonin research by the federal Agency for Healthcare Research and Quality (AHRQ) concluded that the supplement "is not effective in treating most sleep disorders."

While melatonin is no longer seen as advantageous to the broad population of insomniacs, a subset does appear to benefit— those whose insomnia results from delayed sleep phase disorder (DSP), a circadian rhythm disorder in which people don't start to feel sleepy until hours after the traditional bedtime. The AHRQ review found that melatonin enables people with this disorder to fall asleep an average of nearly forty minutes faster than they would with a placebo. I'll discuss melatonin's role in treating DSP in greater detail in Chapter 15.

Melatonin has a short half-life (one or two hours) and does not appear to pose any major health risks when taken for a short time. The most commonly reported side effects are nausea, headache, and dizziness. Its long-term effects are unknown.

Acupuncture

The centuries-old Chinese practice of acupuncture is based on the theory that your physical and mental health depends on a natural flow of energy called *qi* (pronounced "chee") that courses along fourteen pathways known as meridians. When this flow becomes blocked, pain and other health problems (including insomnia) may develop. Acupuncture is intended to relieve this blockage and provide relief.

An acupuncturist inserts fine, sterile needles through the skin along the various meridians. Certain points, particularly those on the legs, arms, wrist, scalp, and ears, are thought to be most effective in treating insomnia. Treatment typically entails three to five thirty-minute sessions per week.

A 2003 review in the *Journal of Advanced Nursing* of eleven studies found that most study participants reported significant sleep improvements. However, the review's author noted that most of the studies were small and based on questionnaires; larger, more meticulous studies in which acupuncture is compared with other insomnia treatments are needed to help assess the therapy's effectiveness.

Hot Baths

A handful of studies have looked at a method known as "passive body heating" to treat insomnia. You take a long, hot bath an hour or two before bedtime, which raises your core body temperature and delays its eventual nighttime drop. Although the effect is not huge, altering the body temperature cycle seems to help some people fall sleep more easily and get more deep sleep. This treatment causes no harm and it feels good, so there's no harm in trying it.

CHAPTER 11

Sleep-Related Breathing Disorders: Snoring and Sleep Apnea

Breathing during sleep is somewhat like a car idling at a stoplight. Ideally, an automobile's engine slows significantly but keeps running smoothly. If it eases up too much, the car may start to sputter a bit or even stop running altogether.

When you sleep, breathing slows, your muscles relax, and your airway narrows slightly, but you continue to inhale and exhale steadily. If for some reason the airway narrows a little too much, you'll start to snore. If the airway narrows completely, breathing may cease altogether, forcing you to gasp for air and temporarily wake up.

Snoring that occurs when the airway is slightly narrowed but still open is referred to as simple, or primary, snoring. While not life-threatening, simple snoring may still be worth treating, since it can severely disrupt your partner's sleep. Complete or near-complete blockage of the airway during sleep is known as obstructive sleep apnea (OSA)—a serious disorder with potentially serious effects on a person's health and quality of life.

In this chapter, we'll look at the causes of and treatments for simple snoring and OSA, as well as a rarer form of sleep apnea known as central sleep apnea (CSA).

Simple Snoring

Forty percent of adults snore, and men are more likely to snore than women. This difference may be due to the protective role played by the hormones progesterone and estrogen; prior to menopause, women snore less than men, but snoring increases among women later in life. Some children snore, but it's more common in adults, especially those who are overweight.

Understanding Snoring

While you sleep, the muscles of your throat relax, and your throat becomes narrower and floppy. This is normal. If the airway narrows too much, airflow becomes turbulent instead of smooth and steady. This makes the walls of the throat begin to vibrate—generally when you breathe in, but also, to a lesser extent, when you breathe out. These vibrations lead to the characteristic sound of snoring. The narrower your airway becomes, the greater the vibration and the louder the snoring.

Causes of snoring include the following:

- **Decreased muscle tone.** Muscle tone decreases as we age, allowing the sides of the throat to close together and the tongue to fall backward into the airway.
- **Obesity.** Being overweight often contributes to snoring, since excess fat in the neck area reduces the width of the air passage.
- **Congestion.** Your nasal passages become inflamed as a response to a cold or allergies, narrowing the air passage and forcing you to inhale even harder to get air into your lungs. Congestion also can occur when you breathe in excessively dry air at night; the mucus in your nose and throat thickens and forms crusts, limiting airflow.

Case History

Elaine, a forty-three-year-old administrator in a health care clinic, came to see me primarily because of her husband's complaints about her loud snoring. Her first consultation also revealed that her husband had noticed that she stopped breathing frequently during the night.

She said that the snoring had worsened as her weight had increased, and she steadily became sleepier during the day. At first she would fall asleep while reading or watching a movie, but now she was dozing off at almost any time—working on her computer, visiting a friend, and once in a public bathroom. She frequently caught herself nodding off while driving but, fortunately, had not had any accidents yet. Her only other medical problem was recurrent migraine headaches.

During an overnight stay in our sleep lab, Elaine was diagnosed with severe obstructive sleep apnea. Her airway was closing off, waking her up fifty-seven times an hour to breathe. With each episode, her blood oxygen level would drop, and then her heart rate would speed up when she awoke. That night, we put her on continuous positive airway pressure (CPAP). Her airway stayed open, no apnea occurred, and she slept continuously.

When she returned for a visit after using CPAP at home for a month, Elaine was a new woman. Her sleepiness was totally gone, and she said she woke up each morning "feeling like the Energizer bunny." Gone was the increased muscle tension she used to feel, and she hadn't had any migraine headaches. She felt so energetic she had started exercising and was committed to losing enough weight to get rid of the OSA and the need for CPAP.

• **Anatomical abnormalities.** Anything that causes airway narrowing can lead to snoring. In the nose, for example, the septum (a three-inch-long partition of bone and cartilage) is often crooked from birth or as the result of blunt trauma during childhood or adulthood. Or the nasal valve—the firm tissue surrounding the passageway in the middle third of your nose that collapses inward slightly when you take a deep breath—may be narrower than normal, making it hard for inhaled air to get by. In the mouth and throat, the tonsils, tongue, uvula (the tissue that hangs down in the back of your throat), and adenoids (a lump of tissue at the back of the nose that contains cells designed to fight infection) may become enlarged and narrow the airway. The soft palate, a muscular flap between the nose and mouth that directs food and air during swallowing or speaking, may become elongated, narrowing the opening from the nose into the throat. A very small or narrow jaw also may contribute to snoring.

- **Alcohol and drugs.** Alcohol and certain prescription medications—such as sedatives for insomnia and anxiety and muscle relaxants for back pain and arthritis—can cause the throat muscles to relax more than usual, resulting in a narrow airway and causing or worsening snoring.

Sleep specialists take all snoring seriously because it may indicate that a person has sleep apnea or is likely to develop it in the near future. It's difficult to distinguish between simple snoring and OSA without studying the person while asleep, so anyone who snores heavily should get a thorough examination of the throat, mouth, palate, tongue, and neck, and may need to undergo a sleep study.

Nonsurgical Treatments for Snoring

There are numerous treatments for snoring that do not entail surgery:

- **Lifestyle changes.** If you're significantly overweight, losing weight often eliminates snoring, since it reduces the amount of fatty tissue in the neck and throat. Quitting smoking, foregoing alcohol in the evening, and avoiding sleeping pills and muscle relaxants may also help.

- **Home solutions.** If you snore only when lying on your back, sewing a tennis or golf ball into the back of your pajamas will prod you to sleep on your side. Another simple solution that helps some snorers is to elevate your head by propping up one end of the bed a few inches. (Extra pillows alone don't provide sufficient support to accomplish this.)
- **Store products.** If congestion is the problem, a humidifier placed on your nightstand may help. Humidifiers tend to make a difference if you live in a hot, desert climate (where the air is naturally dry) or a cold climate (where the indoor air is artificially dry because the heating system produces "dry heat").

    If your snoring results from a narrowed nasal valve, nasal strips or mechanical dilators may work. Nasal strips, which you've probably seen worn by professional athletes, consist of two flat parallel bands of plastic embedded in a special adhesive pad. When placed across the nose, the bands lift the skin upward and outward, pulling open the flexible cartilage walls and widening the nasal valve. Mechanical dilators, usually made of plastic, are inserted just inside the nostril and push outward. Patients whose snoring originates from the mouth and throat won't benefit from these devices.
- **Medication.** If a humidifier doesn't help, snoring caused by congestion may be relieved by a prescription nasal steroid spray such as fluticasone (Flonase), mometasone (Nasonex), or budesonide (Rhinocort) used daily. Avoid over-the-counter spray decongestants (Afrin, Dristan, Neo-Synephrine); their effect diminishes after a few days, excessive use can damage the lining of the nose, and it's easy to become dependent on them.
- **Dental devices.** There are more than forty different devices currently on the market, which fall into two general categories: mandibular (lower jaw) advancing devices or tongue retaining devices. The mandibular advancing devices are used most often. They attach to the upper jaw and force the lower jaw forward, pulling the base of the tongue with it

127

and opening up the airway. The tongue retaining devices use a suction ball at the front of the mouth to hold the tongue forward and open the airway. Dental devices, which are available from dentists, are often effective when worn every night. Some people find them uncomfortable and discontinue use, however.

Surgery

When other remedies prove ineffective and severe snoring persists, surgery is an option. There are several types:

- **Uvulopalatopharyngoplasty (UPPP).** Developed in the 1960s, UPPP was the first surgical procedure for snoring. A surgeon removes the uvula, the tonsils, and a rim of loose tissue at the edge of the soft palate. Recovery is similar to that following a tonsillectomy: You usually have a very painful sore throat for a couple of weeks. The hospital stay usually lasts two days, and you're monitored overnight for potential complications.
- **Laser-assisted uvulopalatoplasty (LAUP).** In 1990, a French physician reported successfully using a type of laser surgery to treat snoring. In this procedure, which is usually done on an outpatient basis under a local anesthetic, an ear, nose, and throat (ENT) specialist uses a laser to shorten the uvula and make small cuts in the soft palate on either side of the uvula. As these nicks heal, the surrounding tissue pulls tighter and stiffens, preventing loose tissue from flapping while you sleep.

  The procedure causes little bleeding. Patients usually have a sore throat for about a week. After five weeks of healing, the treatment may be repeated if snoring persists. Three or four procedures may be needed.

  One important note about LAUP: it can be effective in stopping snoring, but it has not been shown to ease sleep apnea. In fact, undergoing this procedure can be dangerous for people with apnea because it removes the warning signal of this breathing disorder. So it's important to have sleep apnea ruled out by a physician before undergoing LAUP.

- **Somnoplasty.** Also known as radiofrequency tissue volume reduction, this technique was developed by ENTs at Stanford University. In the mid-1990s, the FDA approved this therapy as a treatment for snoring. Somnoplasty is performed on an outpatient basis using a local anesthetic. The doctor delivers radiofrequency waves through the tips of tiny needles inserted into the obstructive tissue to shrink it.

  Somnoplasty only takes a few minutes to perform and doesn't cause bleeding, but it may have to be repeated to achieve results. Although there is typically some swelling immediately following the procedure, posttreatment pain is usually minimal and can be managed with over-the-counter painkillers.

- **Palatal implants.** In 2004, the FDA approved this new procedure (also known as the Pillar procedure) in which up to three matchstick-sized stiffening rods made of polyester material are implanted in the soft palate. The rods help prevent collapse of the palate, limiting obstruction of the back of the throat when a person falls asleep. The procedure, which is done under local anesthesia in an office, is reversible, so if it causes pain or does not work, the rods can be removed—again, under local anesthesia in the office. Sometimes the rods come out on their own, but this does not seem to cause significant discomfort.

  If palatal collapse is the main reason for a patient's snoring, then the procedure may improve symptoms; it has limited benefit when other anatomical problems are involved.

- **Other corrective surgeries.** An operation may be necessary to straighten a deviated septum or remove large tonsils (tonsillectomy). These procedures require general anesthesia and an overnight hospital stay. Removal of enlarged adenoids (adenoidectomy) can be done under local anesthesia on an outpatient basis.

129

Most follow-up studies have found that surgery's long-term success rate is about 50 percent; in some cases, surgery appears successful at first, but snoring returns after a year or so. Palatal implants haven't been performed enough to establish a reliable success rate. If you're considering surgery for snoring, a sleep specialist can review the options in greater detail and help you determine which procedure, if any, is most likely to help you. If you decide on surgery, an ENT specialist will go over success rates, the potential risks, recovery, and the likelihood that you'll need repeat surgery months or years later. Make sure that an evaluation is done to rule out OSA before deciding on any invasive treatment for snoring.

Obstructive Sleep Apnea

Obstructive sleep apnea affects approximately eighteen million adults in the United States and is most frequently seen in overweight men. It was once considered uncommon and often remained undiagnosed. Physicians rarely checked for it except in the stereotypical patient—a sleepy, overweight, middle-aged man who snored. But in 1993, researchers at the University of Wisconsin School of Medicine learned that apnea is more common in both men and women than previously thought. They looked for sleep apnea in six hundred state employees, ages thirty to sixty, as part of a larger sleep study, and were surprised to find that 9 percent of women and 24 percent of men had at least five episodes of airway obstruction per hour. About 4 percent of men and 2 percent of women were estimated to have the full sleep apnea syndrome, which includes abnormal breathing events and daytime sleepiness.

So it's not just overweight men who get OSA. All the things that block the upper airway in simple snoring—such as enlarged tonsils, an elongated uvula, fatty deposits in the airway walls, nasal congestion, or extra floppy tissue at the back of the palate—can cause it. In many cases, people with OSA were born with smaller-than-usual airway openings, which makes obstruction during sleep more likely. Women lose the protective effect of estrogen and progesterone after menopause, and their likelihood of having OSA increases almost to the rate seen in men.

Untreated, OSA can have serious consequences. The relentless daytime fatigue that often results may lead to failed careers, broken marriages, and automobile and workplace accidents. It can even be life-threatening, leading to the development of hypertension, heart failure, and stroke. (A 2005 *New England Journal of Medicine* study found that sleep apnea doubles a person's risk of stroke over a seven-year period.) The disorder is believed to have contributed to the deaths of Grateful Dead guitarist Jerry Garcia and NFL Hall of Famer Reggie White.

Understanding Apnea

As you know, a small amount of airway narrowing at the onset of sleep causes snoring. The more the airway narrows, the harder it is to get an adequate size breath and the greater the effort needed to breath. As breath size gets smaller, blood oxygen levels drop and carbon dioxide builds up. In some cases the airway closes completely and no air gets in at all (see Figure 11.1).

Eventually the increasing effort required to breathe, along with the lack of oxygen and buildup of carbon dioxide, causes the sleeper to awaken and gasp loudly for air. After several large breaths, the blood oxygen and carbon dioxide levels return to normal and the person falls back to sleep, only to repeat the cycle again. Some people with sleep apnea repeat this cycle hundreds of times a night without being fully aware of what is happening.

The repeated awakenings make sleep nonrestful and result in daytime sleepiness. The drops in oxygen and the extra work required to breathe stress the heart and can lead to cardiovascular problems over the long term.

Many people with OSA don't realize how little sleep they're actually getting and assume it's normal to feel lethargic and sleepy all the time. Others wake up after bouts of apnea and have difficulty getting back to sleep; they may reason that insomnia—not a breathing problem—makes them sleepy during the day. The

FIGURE 11.1 Keeping the Airway Open

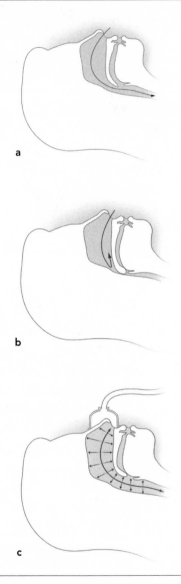

a

b

c

a. Air flows easily through an open airway during normal breathing. b. In obstructive sleep apnea, the airway collapses and blocks airflow. c. Positive airway pressure (PAP) devices keep the airway open, allowing normal airflow.

condition can become even more perilous if a person with apnea is treated with sleeping pills, which can further relax airway muscles or suppress arousal or breathing.

A six-question screening test can help you determine if you need to be tested for sleep apnea. Symptoms and signs include the following:

- **Snoring.** The hallmark of OSA is extremely loud snoring. Bed partners often liken it to a chainsaw or a foghorn, and they notice a pattern of snoring interrupted by periods of silence that end with snorting or gasping sounds. In many cases, the snoring is so irksome that spouses choose to sleep in another room. Not surprisingly, it's often the spouse who forces the person with sleep apnea to seek treatment.
- **Thick neck.** The risk of having OSA rises with increasing neck size, a measure of body weight. Men with a neck circumference of seventeen inches or more and women with a neck circumference of sixteen inches or more are at higher risk. As with snoring, obesity is a major risk factor here, since fatty deposits surrounding the throat expand as people gain weight, narrowing the airway.
- **Hypertension and cardiovascular problems.** The 2003 report from the U.S. National Committee on Prevention, Detection, Evaluation, and Treatment of High Blood Pressure lists sleep apnea as the first of ten identifiable causes of hypertension, and more than half of patients with OSA have it. Other cardiovascular problems are also common; sleep is normally a time of rest for the heart, but sleep apnea forces the heart to work harder every time blood oxygen levels dip and the person wakes up to breathe. OSA patients have a higher risk for stroke, heart attack, heart failure, and arrhythmias (irregular heartbeats), most likely due to the high blood pressure apnea causes.
- **Daytime sleepiness.** People with OSA are excessively sleepy during the day and may fall asleep at unexpected

Screening for Sleep Apnea

This six-question test can help you and your physician determine if you need to be tested for sleep apnea.

Do you snore most nights (more than three times per week)?

    Yes (2)   No (0)

Is your snoring loud (can it be heard through a door or wall)?

    Yes (2)   No (0)

How often are you told that you stop breathing or gasp during sleep?

    Never (0)   Occasionally (3)   Frequently (5)

What is your collar size?

Men

Less than 17 inches (0)   17 inches or greater (5)

Women

Less than 16 inches (0)   16 inches or greater (5)

Have you had, or are you currently being treated for, high blood pressure?

    Yes (2)   No (0)

Do you occasionally doze or fall asleep during the day when you are not busy or active?

    Yes (2)   No (0)

When you are driving or stopped at a light?

    Yes (2)   No (0)

Score

9 points or more: See your physician or a sleep specialist to assess the need for a sleep study.

6–8 points: Uncertain; your physician must use clinical judgment.

Reprinted with permission from Dr. David P. White, Sleep HealthCenters, Newton, Massachusetts.

times. They often describe feeling like they're in a fog all day long.

- **Cognitive problems.** OSA patients report problems with memory, learning, reaction time, and concentration. This is partly due to being too sleepy to pay attention to new things but also may reflect permanent impairment in brain function from oxygen deprivation.
- **Weight gain.** The risk of developing OSA increases as weight goes up. In addition, chronic sleep deprivation causes changes in the levels of the hormones regulating appetite and weight, predisposing a person to weight gain.
- **Diabetes.** Results from the large Sleep Heart Health Study found a strong association between OSA and type 2 diabetes. Animal models suggest that sleep disruption and intermittent drops in oxygen level may cause disruptions in insulin levels and sugar metabolism that lead to diabetes.
- **Other health problems.** People with OSA frequently experience headaches and face an increased risk for depression.

Noninvasive Treatments for OSA

Many of the same treatments for simple snoring are used to treat OSA. Weight loss is the best treatment for weight-related OSA. Sleeping on one's side instead of the back can work for people who only experience OSA in the latter position. Avoidance of alcohol, sedatives, and muscle relaxants is advisable for everyone with OSA. Nasal strips, mechanical dilators, and moisturizing gels and sprays have not been shown to help.

Because weight loss takes time and can be very hard to achieve and maintain, and the other simple measures are usually not sufficient in more severe cases, other treatments are often required.

Positive Airway Pressure (PAP). The first-line therapy for most people with moderate to severe OSA is PAP, an air-pressure device connected by a hose to a mask that covers the nose (see

FIGURE 11.2 Positive Airway Pressure (PAP)

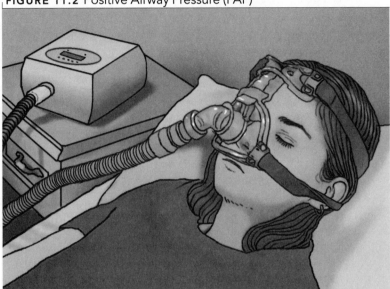

PAP splints open the airway, preventing collapse when muscles around the airway relax during sleep. Pressure is delivered from a bedside air blower through a tube to a mask that covers the nose, allowing the person to sleep normally because breathing is regular and uninterrupted.

Figure 11.2). The air pressure delivered through the mask keeps the airway open, preventing collapse when the muscles relax during sleep and allowing the person to breathe regularly without interruption and sleep normally. The most common form of PAP is continuous positive airway pressure, in which the air pressure stays the same while breathing in and out.

Continuous positive airway pressure was once very cumbersome but has become more comfortable in recent years. Newer models are lighter and quieter, and many offer options such as warmed humidified air (which alleviates nasal congestion, skin dryness, and dry mouth) and a timer that slowly builds up pressure to give you time to adapt and fall asleep more easily. There are also a variety of mask styles, allowing users to find the one that best fits their face and is most comfortable.

People usually try CPAP for the first time in a sleep laboratory, so a technician can adjust the pressure during sleep. Many people take to it without any problem and report that their night in the laboratory is the best night's sleep they've had in years. Others find it difficult at first to breathe out against a constant stream of air and to sleep with their mouth closed, but they usually get used to it with time.

Continuous positive airway pressure generally leads to a great improvement in the amount of time spent in restorative deep sleep, which in turn leads to improved alertness the next day. In many cases, CPAP also reduces or eliminates hypertension. For some people, CPAP is a lifelong treatment.

Other PAP Types. For people who have difficulty exhaling against the pressure of CPAP, a refinement called bi-level PAP (often referred to by the trademarked name BiPAP) may be more tolerable. It delivers air under higher pressure as the sleeper inhales and switches to a lower pressure during exhalation to make it easier to breathe out. The most recent innovation (called AutoPAP) is the inclusion of an internal regulator that moves the pressure up and down, depending on your pressure needs at each particular point in time, rather than keeping it at a fixed setting.

Dental Devices. The same jaw advancing and tongue retaining devices used for simple snoring are the second-line therapy for OSA. These devices are fairly well tolerated and have a 50 to 70 percent success rate for mild to moderate OSA. They are less successful with severe OSA.

These devices are less cumbersome and easier to travel with than CPAP. However, they can cause teeth to shift and initiate problems with the temporomandibular joint (TMJ), so it's important to get the device from a dentist who's trained in managing OSA patients, get regular follow-up, and have a sleep study performed with the device in place to make sure the OSA is eliminated.

Medications. Researchers have tried to develop a medication that stiffens the muscles around the airway and prevents OSA. Unfortunately, there hasn't been much success. One early attempt demonstrated that strychnine stiffens muscles in a test tube, but clearly this poison is of no clinical use. For now, medications are used primarily in conjunction with other treatments.

- **Antidepressants.** Certain antidepressants have a mild positive effect on airway muscle tone and are helpful for a small percentage of people with mild OSA. Two classes of antidepressants are used: tricyclics and selective serotonin reuptake inhibitors.
- **Oxygen.** Supplemental oxygen, administered through a nasal tube, can prevent the drops in blood oxygen that accompany airway collapse. However, oxygen does not prevent the collapse or sleep fragmentation, so it's used in addition to other treatments.
- **Modafinil.** For reasons we don't understand, some people with OSA continue to experience daytime sleepiness even after treatment has eliminated airway obstruction. In 2004 the FDA approved the use of the drug modafinil (Provigil) to counteract this sort of posttreatment sleepiness. The drug, which seems to temporarily inhibit production of neurotransmitters that promote sleep, was originally approved in 1999 to treat sleepiness from narcolepsy. While modafinil can be helpful for people with OSA who have trouble staying alert during the day, it's important to bear in mind that the drug does not address the source of sleep apnea, so it is used in conjunction with other treatments, not in place of them.

Surgical Treatments for OSA

While surgical procedures on many body parts have strong success rates, this is not the case with most surgery for sleep apnea. Although some patients improve, a sizable percentage experience no reduction in symptoms, and some patients' symptoms actually worsen—they have more episodes of apnea after the surgery than they had before.

The unsatisfying success rates of surgery for OSA can be attributed to the fact that surgeons are dealing with a long soft tube of tissue that can collapse at any point—or even at several points—and it's difficult to predict exactly where it might collapse in the future. Surgery corrects collapse at a single spot, so if a collapse subsequently occurs at a different spot (or several different spots), it won't be successful.

That's not to say that surgery is always a bad idea. Next to weight loss, it's one of the only options for a cure. If you have OSA, consult with a sleep specialist to hear about all of your options. Then, if you decide on surgery, find a surgeon who has a lot of experience with these procedures to improve your chances for success.

Types of surgery for OSA include the following:

- **Uvulopalatopharyngoplasty.** When used to treat OSA, UPPP helps about 40 to 45 percent of patients. The rest may need to have further upper airway surgery or use CPAP.
- **Somnoplasty.** Somnoplasty is sometimes used to treat mild sleep apnea when other treatments have not helped. There is limited data supporting its use.
- **Corrective jaw surgery.** Surgery to move the upper or lower jaw forward may enlarge the upper airway for some people with OSA. Centers with specialists in this procedure report success rates of up to 90 percent. However, the procedure requires extensive training and experience for the surgeon, changes the patient's facial appearance and tooth alignment, and has an extensive recovery period.
- **Palatal implants.** Some ENT specialists have started using the implant procedure to treat people whose OSA results from an elongated soft palate. It's not yet clear what percentage of patients benefit or how long improvements last.
- **Tracheostomy.** Tracheostomy, the first surgical treatment used for sleep apnea, is rarely used today due to the success of CPAP and other treatments. The surgeon makes a small

hole through the lower neck into the airway below its point of collapse and inserts a tube. During the day, the tube is plugged; at night, it's opened to allow air to enter, bypassing the obstructed area. Tracheostomy is 100 percent effective, but because of its major detriment to quality of life (including speech difficulties), it is reserved for life-threatening cases or when all other treatments have failed.

Again, consult with your doctor or a sleep specialist about the best treatment for you. The decision depends on the severity of your apnea, the type of symptoms you're having, your overall medical condition, and your personal preferences. I generally recommend that people with moderate to severe OSA start with PAP therapy. If that is not successful, consider a dental appliance and then surgery. For mild OSA, the options are greater and are guided more by personal preference.

Central Sleep Apnea

Central sleep apnea occurs when respiratory centers in the brain fail to send the necessary messages to initiate breathing. Although the airway isn't blocked, the diaphragm and chest muscles stop moving. Falling blood oxygen and rising carbon dioxide levels soon set off an internal alarm, prompting resumption of breathing and often waking the person.

This condition becomes more common as people age, and it's more frequent and severe in those with heart failure, chronic lung disease, or neurological damage. Loud snoring is not a factor. People with CSA are usually aware of waking up during the night and often complain of daytime sleepiness.

Therapy for central sleep apnea usually involves treating the underlying medical condition that has disrupted breathing. For example, if the CSA is caused by heart failure, medications to treat the heart failure may eliminate the CSA. Sometimes CPAP is used, and patients may receive added oxygen. For patients who have CSA only as they begin to fall asleep, a mild sleeping pill may help them go to sleep and stay asleep, solving the breathing problem.

Before deciding on treatment for CSA, it is important to establish the cause. A thorough evaluation, including a sleep study, is warranted. Fortunately, this form of sleep apnea is not common.

CHAPTER 12

Movement Disorders: Restless Legs and Periodic Limb Movements

Normally our arms and legs are mostly still just before and during sleep. Our limbs may twitch once or twice at the onset of sleep—a harmless phenomenon known as hypnic jerks—and we may shift positions during brief awakenings through the night. Otherwise, the deep muscle relaxation accompanying non-REM sleep and the temporary paralysis of REM sleep keep arm and leg movements to a minimum.

People with two neurological sleep disorders—restless legs syndrome (RLS) and periodic limb movement disorder (PLMD)—are an exception to this rule. For them, uncontrollable limb movements are a regular occurrence that can make it impossible to obtain a restful night's sleep. Let's look at the symptoms and treatments for these movement disorders.

Restless Legs Syndrome

This condition is characterized by an uncomfortable urge to move the limbs, accompanied by strange sensations in the lower legs, knees, and occasionally the arms. People perceive and describe the

Sleep-Related Leg Cramps

Leg cramps that wake people up during the night are a common phenomenon, especially among those over fifty. These often-painful cramps are caused by sudden, involuntary contractions of the calf muscles. Occasionally, muscles in the soles of the feet also cramp. The sensation can last a few seconds or up to ten minutes.

We don't know exactly what causes sleep-related leg cramps. In most cases, there doesn't seem to be any specific trigger. Sometimes they seem to be brought on by overexertion of the muscles during the day, prolonged sitting or standing, inappropriate leg positions while sedentary, or dehydration. Electrolyte imbalances, particularly potassium or magnesium, may predispose a person to cramping; such imbalances can be the result of diuretic medications used to treat problems such as heart failure or hypertension. Sleep-related leg cramps also occur more commonly in those with diabetes, peripheral vascular disease, and endocrine disorders.

Often cramping goes away on its own. If it doesn't, straighten the affected leg and flex your foot toward your knee. Grab your toes and pull them upward toward your knee. Usually this works. Applying heat and massaging your leg also may help.

Tactics that may reduce the likelihood of cramps occurring in the first place include drinking plenty of water; stretching and exercising regularly; applying heat to the muscles that have been cramping before bed; and wearing better footwear, such as shoes or inserts with arch support. While potassium, calcium, and vitamin E supplements are often suggested, there's no solid evidence that they're effective unless a deficiency is identified.

Medications are an option for people who experience persistent or severe leg cramps. The malaria drug quinine is effective, but it should be used with caution because it can have unpredictable side effects. There are a number of alternatives, including muscle relaxants and several other drugs such as gabapentin.

sensations of RLS in a variety of ways. Many observe tingling, prickly, itching, and pulling sensations; a few say they feel like they have worms crawling under their skin. Some people find the sensations quite painful.

The sensations—which are different from ordinary leg cramps and the numbness you feel if your leg falls asleep—are typically worst when you lie down to go to sleep at night. They generally begin in the evening, but in some people, they may also occur during daytime periods of inactivity, such as while watching television or flying in a plane. Moving the legs may relieve the discomfort temporarily. People with RLS often develop a variety of coping strategies, such as pacing, doing knee bends, rocking, or stretching the leg muscles, to relieve the symptoms.

About 5 percent of people experience symptoms of RLS at least once a week and 2.7 percent have symptoms twice a week or more, according to a 2005 study of sixteen thousand people in five Western European countries and the United States. Restless legs syndrome is 50 percent more likely to occur in women than men.

Not surprisingly, RLS profoundly affects sleep. The symptoms may compel an individual to get in and out of bed repeatedly, delaying or interrupting sleep. Sleep deprivation from this RLS-induced insomnia often leads to extreme daytime sleepiness. The combination of symptoms and the daytime sleepiness they engender can seriously harm a person's career and social life, since he or she may avoid traveling long distances, attending long meetings, eating at restaurants, and going to movies and concerts. People with RLS are more prone to depression because of the severe impact the disorder can have on their lives. A patient support group, the Restless Legs Syndrome Foundation (rls.org), can provide RLS sufferers with a source for information and the ability to learn from others with the same condition how to adapt and deal with the complications of living with this condition.

Because the symptoms sound bizarre or vague and the need to be constantly mobile seems like nervousness, people with RLS are sometimes mistakenly thought to have psychiatric problems. In

Case History

Maria was a fifty-seven-year-old former schoolteacher who developed progressive kidney disease and symptoms of restless legs syndrome at about the same time. As the kidney disease worsened, so did her RLS symptoms. She was constantly bothered by an itching sensation so severe she had to move around all evening to keep from being driven crazy. She never woke feeling rested and became more and more exhausted with each passing month.

Eventually Maria had a kidney transplant; this took care of her kidney problems but had no affect on her RLS symptoms. When she came to see me, she said she was so tired she rarely left the house. In fact, that morning she hadn't had enough energy to get dressed and arrived in her nightgown and robe, with rollers still in her hair.

A sleep study showed that severe periodic limb movement disorder was disturbing her sleep in addition to the RLS she experienced while awake. I started her on a dopamine agent to treat both.

When Maria returned a month later, she was a changed woman. She was well-dressed, beautifully coiffed, and wide awake. She said her leg discomfort was gone, she slept great at night, and she was no longer sleepy all day. She was feeling so good that she had booked herself on a cruise to see the Panama Canal and had to cut our visit short to catch her boat. I wished her bon voyage as she walked out the door.

the past, they were often misdiagnosed as having hypochondria, manic depression, or a stress–related disorder. Children who have RLS are often incorrectly diagnosed as having attention deficit disorder. Some people report that their symptoms started in adolescence and that adults attributed the problem to growing pains or back trouble. In the large study cited earlier, less than 10 percent of those who told their primary care physician about their symptoms were diagnosed with RLS.

The cause of RLS isn't known, but researchers suspect it's related to a malfunction in the pathways by which the brain controls movement reflexes and sensations. Several such pathways are affected by the brain's transmission of dopamine, a neurotransmitter that helps control muscle activity, natural opiate production, and body iron levels. Increasing the body's level of dopamine, iron, and opiate-like compounds can reduce RLS symptoms. We do know that RLS has a genetic basis, with as many as half of people with the condition noting that other members of their family have similar symptoms. Each child of an affected person has a 50 percent chance of inheriting the condition.

In some people, RLS has been linked to the presence of other medical conditions. Anemia due to iron deficiency may be a contributing factor, while it has also been linked to diabetes, arthritis, kidney failure, and neuropathy (nerve damage). In some people, caffeine, stress, nicotine, fatigue, prolonged exposure to a cold or very warm environment, and certain medications—including antihistamines, antidepressants, or lithium—can exacerbate RLS. Women may find that symptoms flare up during menstruation, pregnancy, or menopause. At least one in four pregnant women experiences restless legs. Although RLS can occur at any time, it often worsens with age and tends to be more common and severe in people over fifty (see Figure 12.1).

There is no single diagnostic test for RLS, and standard neurological examinations often reveal no abnormality. Because of its unique symptoms—the strange sensations and the almost irresistible need to move the affected limb—a doctor's diagnosis is made based on the individual's description of symptoms. The doctor will also review the patient's medical history and family history; conduct a physical examination; and order routine blood tests to check for anemia, iron or vitamin deficiency, diabetes, or kidney problems.

FIGURE 12.1 Prevalence of Restless Legs Syndrome by Age

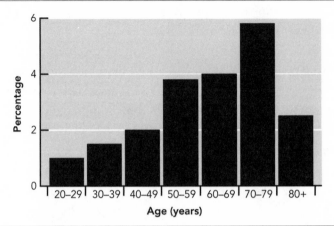

Age (years)

RLS can occur at any age, but it tends to be more common and severe in people over fifty.   Source: Adapted from R. P. Allen, et al., "Restless Legs Syndrome Prevalence and Impact." *Archives of Internal Medicine* 165, 2005: 1286–92.

Treating RLS

Treatment of RLS is aimed at controlling the often-debilitating sensations. The first approach is to look for factors that might be contributing to the symptoms. When RLS is linked to iron deficiency anemia, doctors prescribe iron supplements. Lifestyle changes, such as following a balanced diet that contains iron and eliminating or cutting down on caffeine, alcohol, and cigarette smoking, may also help. For mild cases, exercising (which increases the body's production of natural opiates), stretching or massaging your legs, applying heat or ice packs, or taking a hot bath may bring relief. Over-the-counter pain relievers such as aspirin and ibuprofen benefit some people.

If these treatments don't work, medications from one of several drug classes may be prescribed (see Table 12.1). People often need to try several drugs before finding one that works for them. The medications do not cure RLS; they manage the symptoms and are usually needed on a permanent basis.

- **Dopamine agents.** Several drugs that ease the tremors of Parkinson's disease also reduce the frequency of RLS

TABLE 12.1 Medications for Movement Disorders

Category	Generic Name	Brand Name	Comments
Benzodiazepines	Clonazepam	Klonopin	Side effects may include clumsiness or unsteadiness, dizziness, light-headedness, daytime drowsiness, and headache. Not to be used by people with untreated sleep apnea or other breathing difficulties; not to be used with alcohol or other depressants. May be habit forming. Withdrawal symptoms may occur if stopped abruptly.
	Diazepam	Valium	
	Temazepam	Restoril	
Dopamine agents	Bromocriptine	Parlodel	Side effects may include abnormal movements, depression, mental changes, nausea, and dizziness. Certain drugs in this class should not be used if there is sensitivity to ergotic drugs, in cases of hypertension or glaucoma, or with monoamine oxidase inhibitors (MAOIs).
	Levodopa/ carbidopa	Sinemet	
	Pergolide	Permax	
	Pramipexole	Mirapex	
	Ropinirole*	Requip	
Opiates	Oxycodone	Oxycontin	Side effects may include depressed breathing and circulation, dizziness or light-headedness, next-day sedation, constipation, nausea, and vomiting. There is a risk of addiction. Not to be used by persons with untreated sleep apnea; not to be used with alcohol or other depressants.
	Propoxyphene	Darvon	
	Codeine	Generic only	
	Methadone	Dolophine Methadose	
Anticonvulsants	Carbamazepine	Tegretol	Side effects may include unsteadiness, vision problems, body aches, and congestion. Tegretol may decrease the number of blood cells produced.
	Gabapentin	Neurontin	
	Valproic acid	Depakene	

*Ropinirole is FDA approved to treat restless legs syndrome. Other medications in this chart are not approved to treat RLS or PLMD, but physicians have found that they help people with these conditions.

symptoms. These include levodopa/carbidopa (Sinemet), pergolide (Permax), pramipexole (Mirapex), bromocriptine (Parlodel), and ropinirole (Requip). The brain converts these drugs into dopamine, which seems to limit unwanted muscle sensations and movement.

In 2005, Requip became the first drug approved by the FDA to treat RLS; the others are prescribed off-label. The most common side effects from dopamine agents are daytime drowsiness, nausea, dizziness, and digestive problems.

Note that while the drugs used to treat RLS are the same as those used for Parkinson's disease, people with RLS are no more likely to develop Parkinson's disease than other individuals.

- **Benzodiazepines.** People with mild RLS may be prescribed sleep aids such as clonazepam (Klonopin) or temazepam (Restoril). These drugs don't reduce leg sensations or movements, but they may enable a person to sleep through them. Although many people who take benzodiazepines for insomnia develop a tolerance after a few weeks, this doesn't seem to happen when such drugs are taken for RLS.

- **Opioids.** Because of the potential for addiction when these drugs are misused, physicians are reluctant to treat sleep disturbances with medications derived from opium such as propoxyphene (Darvon), codeine, methadone, and oxycodone (Oxycontin). However, when all other medications have failed, these drugs can be effective in eliminating RLS symptoms. The opiates decrease the discomfort of RLS and, for some patients, dramatically reduce leg movements at night. When taken properly, they may provide long-term benefit with little risk of addiction. Side effects may include nausea, constipation, and next-day sedation.

- **Anticonvulsants.** These medicines, which include gabapentin (Neurontin) and carbamazepine (Tegretol), are primarily used for patients whose RLS symptoms are painful. Side effects may include unsteadiness, vision problems, body aches, and congestion.

Periodic Limb Movement Disorder

Like RLS, periodic limb movement disorder is a neurological condition that affects the legs and arms and your ability to sleep at night. During the night, leg muscles involuntarily contract, which causes kicking or jerking movements, typically every twenty to forty seconds. The same movement (involving the hip, knee, or ankle) may be repeated hundreds of times.

There are two key differences between RLS and PLMD:

- RLS occurs while you're awake; PLMD occurs while you're asleep.
- The movements of RLS are a voluntary response to unpleasant sensations; the movements of PLMD are involuntary (that is, not consciously controlled).

Episodes of PLMD may last only a few minutes or they may continue for hours, with intervals of sound sleep in between. They usually don't occur continuously throughout the night, but instead cluster in the first half of the night and arise predominantly in non-REM sleep.

Even though people with PLMD are usually unaware of their limb movements, sleep can still be affected. Instead of proceeding smoothly through all the sleep stages in regular cycles, they awaken for a few seconds at a time (generally without realizing it) and frequently skip back to the lighter stages of sleep. Unless a bed partner complains, people with PLMD are often oblivious to the movements and may wake up baffled at why they feel exhausted despite getting what they thought was a full night's rest.

What usually brings people with PLMD to my office are complaints from a partner whose sleep is being disrupted. Often an aggrieved spouse drags the patient in, saying that he or she is being repeatedly kicked during the night or that constant jerking of the bed makes it impossible to sleep. As you can imagine, these problems can drive people into different bedrooms and strain marriages. In other cases, people with the disorder come in complaining of daytime sleepiness.

PLMD's cause is still unknown. As with RLS, it probably stems from a malfunction of the central nervous system and may be related to the neurotransmitter dopamine. PLMD is rare in people under thirty but becomes more common as people age. One-third of people age fifty to sixty-five and almost half of people over sixty-five have PLMD.

Although RLS and PLMD are two separate disorders, they do overlap. Nearly everyone with RLS also has PLMD. However, people with PLMD often do not have RLS.

Many of the same factors that raise a person's risk for RLS may also contribute to or worsen PLMD, such as certain beverages, medications, and illnesses. In particular, people with kidney disease and narcolepsy have an elevated risk for PLMD.

Treating PLMD

PLMD does not need to be treated if it doesn't lead to daytime sleepiness or disrupt a partner's sleep. When these problems do occur, the same medications used to treat RLS—dopamine agents, benzodiazepines, opioids, and anticonvulsants—often control or eliminate symptoms.

CHAPTER 13

Narcolepsy

Narcolepsy is a debilitating disorder in which people experience overwhelming waves of drowsiness that may strike at any hour of the day, putting them to sleep during conversations, meetings, meals, and other ordinary activities. In this respect, narcolepsy can be considered the opposite of insomnia—the yin to insomnia's yang—since an insomniac has trouble falling asleep and a narcoleptic has trouble staying awake. But as you'll see, there's much more to narcolepsy, in terms of its unique symptoms and what it tells us about how our bodies make the transition from sleep to wakefulness.

Causes of Narcolepsy

Narcolepsy is a chronic central nervous system disorder in which the brain does not properly regulate the daily cycle of sleep and wakefulness. This malfunction leads to abnormalities in REM sleep and in the timing of sleep and wakefulness. Instead of occurring normally—after a steady progression through the other stages of sleep—REM sleep intrudes at unusual and unwelcome times, such as when a person lies down for a nap, moments after sleep begins, or even in the midst of daytime activities. Currently, there is no cure.

The Flip-Switch Theory of Sleep

Research on narcolepsy has led to a better understanding of the brain's sleep/wake mechanisms. We now understand that several brain systems are involved in regulating sleep and wakefulness. Some brain centers and pathways stimulate the entire brain to wakefulness; others promote falling asleep. Hypocretin's role seems to be to keep a person asleep or awake for long periods of time and make sure the different aspects of each sleep stage occur only during the appropriate stage.

Dr. Clifford Saper of Harvard Medical School, a researcher who has studied narcolepsy, describes the sleep/wake process as a "flip-switch" system (see Figure 13.1). We don't slowly become aware of waking up or falling asleep. Rather, the process happens very quickly, then stabilizes in the new state.

Hypocretin seems to be involved in regulating when the flip between states occurs and keeping you in the new state. In narcolepsy, where there is little or no hypocretin, people flip back and forth between sleep and wakefulness frequently. They fall asleep more often during the day and wake up frequently at night. Features normally confined to REM sleep, such as muscle paralysis and dreaming, can occur during wakefulness or during the transition from sleep to wakefulness.

About one in two thousand people has narcolepsy. The disorder affects both sexes equally, and it has a genetic component; having a close relative with narcolepsy makes a person twenty to forty times more likely to have it. Narcolepsy usually becomes apparent during adolescence or young adulthood, although symptoms sometimes appear in early childhood or middle age.

In the late 1990s, researchers discovered that many cases of narcolepsy result from the lack of a brain chemical called hypocretin (also sometimes called orexin) that normally maintains arousal and helps regulate sleep. Individuals with narcolepsy appear to lose the cells that make hypocretin. It's unclear why this occurs; it may be that narcolepsy is an autoimmune disease, like lupus or multi-

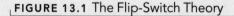

FIGURE 13.1 The Flip-Switch Theory

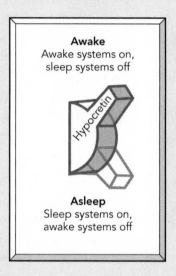

The sleep/wake process can be likened to a flip-switch system in which a chemical in the brain called hypocretin regulates when the flip between wakefulness and sleep occurs. Source: Adapted from C. B. Saper et al., "Hypothalamic Regulation of Sleep and Circadian Rhythyms," *Nature* 437, 2005: 1257–63.

ple sclerosis, in which the body's own immune cells destroy necessary structures. Researchers have identified the specific gene responsible for making hypocretin and the site in the body where it is made. The improved understanding of hypocretin's role in narcolepsy may one day lead to a cure.

Symptoms of Narcolepsy

Narcolepsy has five main symptoms:

- Excessive daytime sleepiness
- Cataplexy

- Sleep paralysis
- Hallucinations
- Insomnia and fragmented sleep

Most people with the disorder have more than one symptom, and some experience all five.

Excessive Daytime Sleepiness

This is usually the first symptom to appear, and everyone with narcolepsy has it. This isn't mild drowsiness that causes a yawn or two; individuals with narcolepsy feel an overwhelming and recurring need to sleep at times when they want to be awake. Even if they struggle to fend it off, they often fall asleep, usually for five to ten minutes.

These unwanted sleep episodes—sometimes referred to as sleep attacks because they come on so quickly and are so powerful—may occur several times a day. Most often they occur while the person is sitting or standing. Some people can sense when an attack is imminent, but others find that they occur without warning. These sleep attacks occur on top of a near-constant feeling of tiredness.

Most sleep attacks are uneventful—the person falls asleep and wakes up a few minutes later feeling temporarily rested. If REM sleep and dreaming occur immediately, the individual sometimes makes conversation in response to the dream instead of the actual situation.

Cataplexy

More than half of people with narcolepsy experience cataplexy—brief episodes of sudden loss of muscle function while awake. Cataplexy is an aspect of REM malfunction; it occurs when the brain mechanism that paralyzes muscles during REM sleep becomes activated during the day. Cataplexy can set in several years after daytime sleepiness first appears or be the disorder's first symptom.

Episodes are typically brought on by laughing and anger or other strong emotion. In mild cases, the person's knees may buckle, or the muscles of the jaw or neck may become weak and difficult to control. In severe cases, the muscles become completely paralyzed, and the person may fall to the ground. These falls occur slowly, so they rarely cause injuries. The person is usually fully awake and aware of what's going on but is unable to talk and appears to be asleep. Although cataplexy sometimes leads to sleep, usually the person recovers spontaneously after several seconds or minutes.

Sleep Paralysis

About 50 to 60 percent of people with narcolepsy experience sleep paralysis—being unable to talk or move for several minutes when falling asleep or waking up. Like cataplexy, sleep paralysis results from the muscle lockdown that normally occurs during REM sleep intruding into wakefulness. It can be very frightening to people the first time, since they may fear they won't be able to breathe. In reality, breathing is not affected, so these episodes are less alarming in subsequent occurrences.

Hypnagogic Hallucinations

An estimated 50 to 60 percent of narcoleptics experience hypnagogic hallucinations—vivid and often frightening images, sounds, or physical sensations from dreams that occur just as they are falling asleep or awakening and that are difficult to distinguish from reality. Again, this symptom results from an activity that would normally occur during REM sleep (dreaming) arising during wakefulness.

Like nightmares, hypnagogic hallucinations often have dangerous themes, such as being pursued or the house burning. These episodes often occur simultaneously with sleep paralysis, adding to their frightfulness. If not recognized as a narcolepsy symptom, hypnagogic hallucinations can be mistaken for a sign of mental illness.

Insomnia and Fragmented Sleep

Ironically, despite falling asleep multiple times during the day, people with narcolepsy typically sleep very poorly at night. They

Case History

By the time twenty-three-year-old Kim came to see me, she had suffered from problems with excessive sleepiness for many years. She recalled difficulty staying awake during class in high school. In college, she was frequently embarrassed when she fell asleep during class, even when she sat directly in front of her professor to help stay awake. Kim also often had vivid, frightening dreams just as she was falling asleep. She fell asleep quickly and stayed asleep, but even though she slept about seven hours a night, she still had trouble staying awake during the daytime.

When we first met, Kim had completed graduate school and was getting ready to begin a teaching job, but she was worried about her commute because she often got drowsy when driving, especially in the morning. I learned that sleepiness ran in her family; she had a grandfather who was always falling asleep, but he had never been evaluated for a sleep disorder. Kim also told me she was prone to depression and had been on antidepressant medication since college.

Kim's uncontrollable sleepiness and her vivid dreams suggested that she had narcolepsy. However, she didn't have any

often have difficulty falling asleep and wake up frequently. While asleep, they do not follow the typical REM/non–REM cycle; REM sleep can happen immediately or at any time.

Other Symptoms

About half of people with narcolepsy experience automatic behavior—episodes lasting several minutes or more during which they perform routine tasks (often incorrectly) without being fully aware of what they are doing. Examples include putting a roast in the dishwasher, driving past an intended exit on the highway, or writing off the edge of a page. Other occasional narcolepsy symp-

symptoms of muscle weakness, which would have clinched the diagnosis.

To evaluate the problem, she stayed overnight at our sleep clinic and the next day took the multiple sleep latency test (MSLT), which monitors how long it takes a person to fall asleep during five daytime nap opportunities. Aside from falling asleep very quickly (taking an average of less than three minutes to nod off with each nap opportunity), the overnight sleep study showed no sleep fragmentation that could account for Kim's sleepiness. She also went into REM sleep within fifteen minutes on two of the naps. Taken altogether, this pattern was consistent with narcolepsy.

To manage Kim's sleepiness, I prescribed a series of stimulant medications. She did best with modafinil (Provigil). A single dose in the morning kept her alert throughout the day and eliminated her drowsiness while driving. Her sleepiness was not totally eliminated—if she sat down with nothing to do, she could easily nod off—but she functioned well at her new job and could engage in any activity she wanted. Her mood also improved.

toms include blurred vision, difficulty with memory or concentrating, and migraine headaches.

Diagnosis

Diagnosis of narcolepsy typically begins with a doctor having you describe your symptoms, taking a medical history, and doing a physical exam. If you have both excessive daytime sleepiness and cataplexy, there's a very good chance that you have narcolepsy. If daytime sleepiness and one of the other symptoms are present (without cataplexy), it could be narcolepsy, but the symptoms might also be caused by another health problem, such as sleep apnea. When narcolepsy seems likely, the doctor may refer you to a sleep specialist, who will evaluate your sleep during the day and at night.

Nighttime sleep is evaluated first with an overnight sleep study in which polysomnography is used to measure brain waves and body movements (Chapter 18 describes the process in detail). Compared to normal sleepers, people with narcolepsy reach REM more quickly, have more total REM episodes, and have REM sleep at irregular times (not within ninety-minute sleep cycles). They may also wake up more often. Figure 13.2 shows how a narcoleptic's sleep compares with a non-narcoleptic's over twenty-four hours.

After the night study, daytime sleep is evaluated by the multiple sleep latency test. This test consists of five twenty-minute opportunities to nap, which are offered every two hours through-

FIGURE 13.2 Comparison of Sleep Patterns in Normal Sleepers and Narcoleptics

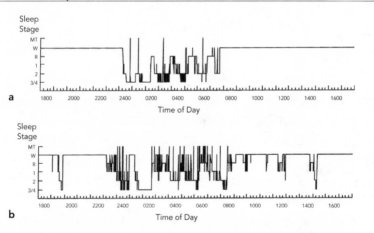

As these hypnograms show, compared to (a) a healthy sleeper, (b) a narcoleptic has more fragmented sleep, experiences frequent daytime sleep periods, and enters REM sleep more quickly and frequently. (Times are given per the military twenty-four-hour clock.) Source: Adapted from Thomas Roth, et al., "Experimental Sleep Fragmentation," *Sleep* 17, 1994: 438–43. Adapted by permission of the American Academy of Sleep Medicine.

out the day. Patients with narcolepsy fall asleep in approximately five minutes or less on average for all naps and move into REM sleep during at least two of the five. Normal, well-rested sleepers average about twelve to fourteen minutes or longer to fall asleep on the daytime naps and don't fall into REM sleep within the twenty minutes.

In cases where the diagnosis cannot be established because test results are inconclusive, it's possible to measure brain levels of hypocretin. This requires a spinal tap, an uncomfortable procedure in which a small needle is passed into the fluid-filled sac surrounding the spinal cord and a small amount of fluid is removed. Narcoleptics have low levels of hypocretin or none at all. Researchers are working on a simple blood test to measure hypocretin, but this is not yet available.

In cases where sleep attacks and cataplexy coexist and occur frequently, narcolepsy is diagnosed quickly. Less obvious cases often take years of symptoms and multiple visits to physicians before the correct diagnosis is made. Narcolepsy is often misdiagnosed as depression, thyroid disorder, chronic fatigue syndrome, and even schizophrenia.

Treatment

Since there is no cure, treatment of narcolepsy is geared toward improving wakefulness during the day and preventing REM-related symptoms. Three types of medications are used: stimulants, antidepressants, and anticataplectics (see Table 13.1). The goal is to approach normal alertness while minimizing side effects and disruptions to daily activities.

- **Stimulants.** The stimulant medications that have been around the longest are related to amphetamines and include methylphenidate (Ritalin, Metadate, Concerta) and dextroamphetamine (Dexedrine, Adderall). These medicines counteract sleep attacks and drowsiness. Common side effects include headaches, irritability, nervousness, insomnia,

TABLE 13.1 Medications for Narcolepsy

Category	Generic Name	Brand Name	Use	Comments
Stimulants I	Dextroamphetamine	Dexedrine, Adderall	To counter daytime sleepiness	Side effects may include nervousness, insomnia, loss of appetite, nausea, dizziness, irregular heartbeat, headaches, changes in blood pressure and pulse, and weight loss. There is a potential for abuse.
	Methylphenidate	Ritalin, Metadate, Concerta		
				Dextroamphetamine and methylphenidate should not be used with monoamine oxidase inhibitors (MAOIs) or in cases of glaucoma.
Stimulants II	Modafinil*	Provigil	To counter daytime sleepiness	Side effects may include anxiety, headache, nausea, nervousness, and insomnia. There is less potential for abuse than with other stimulants.
Tricyclic antidepressants	Clomipramine	Anafranil	To prevent cataplexy and other REM-related symptoms	Side effects may include dizziness, dry mouth, blurred vision, weight gain, constipation, trouble urinating, drowsiness, and disturbance of heart rhythm. Should not be used with MAOIs or during immediate recovery from a heart attack.
	Desipramine	Norpramin		
	Imipramine	Tofranil		
	Protriptyline	Vivactil		
SSRI antidepressants	Fluoxetine	Prozac	To prevent cataplexy and other REM-related symptoms	Side effects may include nausea, dry mouth, headache, loss of appetite, nervousness, diarrhea or constipation, sweating, and sexual problems. Should not be used with MAOIs.
	Paroxetine	Paxil		
	Sertraline	Zoloft		

TABLE 13.1 Medications for Narcolepsy, *continued*

Category	Generic Name	Brand Name	Use	Comments
Anticataplectic	Sodium oxybate*	Xyrem	To prevent cataplexy and improve nighttime sleep	Side effects may include abdominal pain, chills, dizziness, abnormal dreams, drowsiness, and stomach discomfort. Must be taken at bedtime and again during the middle of the night. There is a potential for abuse.

*Modafinil and sodium oxybate are FDA approved to treat narcolepsy symptoms. Other medications in this chart are not approved for this use, but physicians have found that they often help people with narcolepsy.

irregular heartbeat, and mood changes, and there is also a potential for abuse. Another stimulant, pemoline (Cylert), was taken off the market in 2005 because of problems with liver damage.

Modafinil (Provigil), a once-a-day medication to promote wakefulness, received FDA approval for treating daytime sleepiness in 1998. This medication has a different mechanism of action than the older stimulants and is less potent, so there's less concern about its misuse or abuse. Modafinil is quickly becoming the first-line therapy because it has fewer side effects.

- **Antidepressants.** Antidepressants that suppress REM sleep can prevent cataplexy, sleep paralysis, and hypnagogic hallucinations. Two classes are used: selective serotonin reuptake inhibitors (SSRIs) and tricyclics. Side effects vary depending on the drug but may include drowsiness, sexual dysfunction, and lowered blood pressure.
- **Xyrem.** Sodium oxybate (Xyrem), also known as gamma-hydroxybutyrate (GHB), gained FDA approval in 2002 to treat cataplexy caused by narcolepsy. It's the only drug available in its class (anticataplectics). This medication is

effective in decreasing the number of cataplexy episodes and may improve nighttime sleep and reduce daytime sleepiness as well. Xyrem's effects do not last long, so it must be taken at bedtime and again during the middle of the night.

Xyrem is tightly regulated because of its potential for misuse; it can cause daytime amnesia and has been associated with criminal acts such as date rape. Abuse can lead to dependence and severe withdrawal symptoms. When used correctly, side effects may include confusion, depression, nausea, vomiting, dizziness, headache, bed-wetting, and sleepwalking.

Along with drug treatment, several elements of sleep hygiene may help reduce narcolepsy symptoms. These include avoiding caffeine, nicotine, and alcohol in the late afternoon or evening; exercising regularly; establishing a routine time for going to bed and getting up and following it regularly; and getting enough nighttime sleep.

Planned daytime naps may help control excessive sleepiness and sleep attacks. Some people take several twenty- to thirty-minute naps; others prefer a single afternoon nap lasting eighty to ninety minutes. Either way, it's important to allow ten minutes or so afterward to wake up fully before resuming activity.

Psychological counseling may be helpful in cases where narcolepsy interferes with relationships, causes problems with self-esteem, or triggers mental health issues. Support groups (such as the Narcolepsy Network) also can be extremely beneficial, since they put people in touch with others who are coping with similar situations.

Living with Narcolepsy

Undiagnosed and untreated, narcolepsy often takes a heavy toll. Younger people are apt to have trouble performing well in school. Adults may have problems getting and keeping jobs. At any age, untreated narcolepsy can strain relationships with family members and make it hard to make and maintain platonic and romantic relationships. In addition, people with untreated narcolepsy are at increased risk for injuries resulting from motor vehicle or job-related accidents.

When the disorder is recognized and treated, people with narcolepsy can lead fruitful lives. Finding the best drug regimen will reduce daytime sleepiness, the number of unwanted sleep episodes, and other symptoms. In addition, parents, teachers, employers, and friends and family can be made aware of the disorder, so the person's symptoms aren't mistaken for indifference, laziness, lack of motivation, or mental illness. With the use of stimulant medication, it's usually safe for the person to drive. Certain compromises may be necessary—such as finding a job that keeps the person active, avoiding long drives, and skipping sedentary social activities such as movies and plays—but there's no reason people with narcolepsy can't have successful careers and enjoyable personal lives.

CHAPTER 14

Parasomnias: Sleepwalking and Other Unusual Behaviors

For most people, sleep is generally an uneventful part of life; the question "How'd you sleep?" can often be answered with a one-word reply ("Okay"). But for people with any of the unusual sleep disorders known as parasomnias, sleep is anything but dull. They may sit up and let out piercing screams, or kick and punch their bed partner during vivid nightmares. Or they get up out of bed and wander—perhaps to the refrigerator for a snack or right out the front door.

Sleep doctors group parasomnias by the phase of sleep during which they're most likely to occur. There are two main groups: disorders that occur primarily during deep (or non-REM) sleep, and those that occur during REM sleep. We'll look at these two groups and then conclude with two problems—sleep-related eating disorders and bruxism—that don't fall neatly into either category.

Deep Sleep Parasomnias

Non-REM parasomnias include sleepwalking, sleep terrors, and confusional arousals. These three disorders are distinct, but they share several features:

- They begin during the first third of the night (when we get the most deep sleep).
- They occur most commonly in children.
- They usually disappear during adolescence without intervention but may persist into adulthood or even arise later in life.
- They have a genetic basis, often occurring in several generations of the same family.
- They generally don't have serious health consequences and do not require treatment.
- They can be treated successfully with behavioral therapies or sleeping pills in cases where the person's health or safety is endangered.

Sleepwalking

Sleepwalking, or somnambulism, is a phenomenon in which the brain remains partially asleep but the body is still capable of movement. Sometimes sleepwalkers engage in a simple activity, such as pacing back and forth by the bed, but they may also carry out complex actions, such as getting dressed, cleaning the kitchen, or leaving the residence. Scientists used to believe that sleepwalkers were acting out dreams, but this view was discredited with the discovery in 1965 that sleepwalking begins during deep sleep, not REM sleep (when most dreaming occurs).

Episodes usually occur one to two hours after going to sleep. Most last fifteen minutes or less, but they can go on for an hour more. Sleepwalkers' eyes are open and they can see what they're doing, but they wear a blank expression, do not respond to their name or conversation, and generally lack the sense of awareness we associate with wakefulness. Movements tend to be clumsy, prompting some sleepwalkers to trip over furniture or knock over objects. Even so, some sleepwalkers are capable of complex behavior, such as getting into and starting a car.

Because somnambulists are in deep sleep, they are usually difficult to rouse and if awakened are usually confused about where they are and what they were doing. Most episodes end with sleepwalkers going back to bed on their own and returning to normal sleep. (Children often crawl into their parents' bed.) Sleepwalkers usually have no memory of the episode in the morning.

Unfortunately, not all episodes end so smoothly. A small percentage of sleepwalkers suffer injuries when they trip and fall, walk through glass, or attempt to drive. There are also rare reports of somnambulists committing violent crimes, such as assault and murder.

Sleepwalking is most common in school-age children, with up to 15 percent of kids ages five to twelve walking in their sleep at least once, and 4 percent having frequent episodes. The condition is more common in boys than girls. Childhood somnabulism is believed to result from immaturity in the brain's regulation of sleep/wake cycles. The entire brain normally wakes up at the same time; with sleepwalkers, the part responsible for mobility wakes up in response to an arousal, but the part responsible for awareness and cognition stays asleep. Most children outgrow the symptoms by adolescence as their nervous systems develop.

About 1 percent of adults sleepwalk. It can be triggered by sleep disorders that fragment sleep, sleep deprivation, stress, anxiety, or medical conditions such as epilepsy. Heavy consumption of alcohol may also be a contributing factor.

For children who sleepwalk, treatment isn't usually necessary, since they will eventually outgrow the disorder. During an episode, parents should gently guide the child back to bed, offering comforting statements such as, "It's OK, you're going back to bed." There's no need to wake the child up.

Treatment for grown-ups depends on how likely they are to hurt themselves. This assessment is based on factors such as the frequency of events, whether the person leaves the bedroom, whether the bedroom is potentially dangerous (such as on the third floor or with a glass door), whether there's someone else nearby to direct him or her back to bed, and the individual's health and age. As long as the sleepwalker returns to bed without incident, treatment may not be necessary.

Treatment is advisable in cases where people have injured themselves or seem likely to. Behavioral therapies aimed at promoting relaxation often reduce or eliminate episodes. In particular, self-hypnosis—a technique that can be learned from a trained counselor in six sessions and then practiced at home before bedtime—is often effective.

Prescription sleep medications such as benzodiazepines may help, because they reduce the likelihood of a person having a partial awakening. Tricyclic antidepressants also help in some cases, probably for the same reason.

Whether or not treatment is needed, it's a good idea to take precautions to make the sleepwalker's bedroom and house as safe as possible, such as removing sharp or breakable objects, locking doors, putting heavy drapes in front of windows or glass doors, and hiding car keys at night.

Sleep Terrors

Sleep terrors (also known as night terrors) are severe attacks of fear or panic during sleep. An episode is a dramatic sight: the individual suddenly sits up in bed with a terrified expression and lets out an intense, spine-chilling scream. Screams are often accompanied by a racing pulse, rapid breathing, widened pupils, and profuse sweating.

Sleep terrors usually arise during the first third of the night, but they can occur at any time of night and during daytime naps. They generally last from thirty seconds to a few minutes. After the spell is over, the person often goes back to sleep and later does not remember what happened.

One odd aspect of sleep terrors is that the person experiencing an episode is inconsolable—soothing words from family members do not make the person feel any better. For this reason, those in the vicinity should just let the episode run its course.

If the person wakes up anyway, he or she may report temporary breathing difficulty. When prompted, memory often consists of a still image rather than a series of dreamlike images. This image is often frightening, such as a monster, animal, or person poised to kill. It may also be breathing related, such as a pile of rocks on the chest.

Up to 6 percent of children have recurrent sleep terrors, and the incidence in boys and girls is about the same. In most cases, children outgrow the episodes without treatment by adolescence; prevalence in adults is less than 1 percent.

The cause of sleep terrors is unknown. In some instances, episodes are triggered by environmental noises, a partner climbing into bed, or other stimuli. Sleep fragmentation disorders and sleep deprivation may also be a factor.

Despite their frightening nature, sleep terrors generally have no negative health or emotional effects, and treatment is not usually warranted. However, it may be necessary if episodes occur frequently (especially enough to disrupt a bed partner's sleep), show no signs of abating, and lead to anxiety that sparks insomnia, or if the person acts aggressively, such as bolting out of bed to escape or thrashing about as if to fight someone off. Therapy typically consists of medications (benzodiazepines and tricyclic antidepressants) and relaxation techniques (self-hypnosis and guided imagery).

Confusional Arousals

Confusional arousals are events in which sleepers sit up in bed and act extremely disoriented and confused. They don't respond to other people's voices and may do seemingly nonsensical things, such as picking up a shoe and speaking into it as though it were a telephone. They may also moan or mumble incomprehensibly. Occasionally, particularly after a forced awakening, the behavior can be violent, with the person demanding to be left alone to sleep. However, unlike sleep terrors, confusional arousals do not elicit screams; the predominant feature is confusion, not fright.

Confusional arousals are sometimes referred to as "sleep drunkenness" because the foggy behavior resembles intoxication. However, they are not alcohol related. Like sleep terrors, confusional arousals generally last from thirty seconds to a few minutes, after which the person goes back to sleep and usually has no memory of the event. They generally happen early in the night but can also occur closer to one's normal wake-up time. There are usually no negative health or emotional consequences.

Confusional arousals occur most often in children under five and almost always cease by adolescence. They occur in adulthood less commonly than sleepwalking and sleep terrors. Very rarely, people having confusional arousals may hurt themselves or others. In such cases, treatment with sleeping pills may be warranted.

REM Parasomnias

The two major REM parasomnias are REM sleep behavior disorder and nightmares.

REM Sleep Behavior Disorder

Most people make subtle twitching movements during REM sleep, but a temporary muscle paralysis prevents larger movements. In some people, this paralysis evaporates during the night, freeing them to act out dreams. Most often they shout and kick or punch perceived aggressors; they may even jump out of bed onto the floor or up on a table. Such episodes can be dangerous to people experiencing them as well as their bed partners; injuries such as black eyes and bruised ribs are not uncommon.

This phenomenon—known as REM sleep behavior disorder (RBD)—was identified in the 1980s. It's estimated to occur in one in two hundred people (0.5 percent). Nine out of ten people who have it are men. The disorder nearly always arises after age fifty, but there are occasional reports of it occurring in younger adults and children.

Episodes tend to arise in the latter half of the night, when the highest percentage of REM sleep occurs. Typically, the person is experiencing a frightening dream in which he or she feels threatened, such as by an animal, a burglar, or an enemy soldier. In the dream, the person either flees the aggressor or fights back. RBD can lead to a painfully ironic situation in which people are simultaneously defending their partners in their dream and hurting those partners in reality.

RBD can have devastating effects on relationships. Wives have come to my office reporting they are afraid to sleep in the same room with their husbands because they are worried about getting hurt.

Most often, episodes end when the spouse wakes the dreamer by shouting or shaking him or her. Unlike parasomnias that occur during deep sleep, the person isn't confused or disoriented—instead, he or she usually wakes up quickly and can vividly recall the dream in detail. To the person experiencing the episode, it feels like an ordinary nightmare. People who sleep through the night after an RBD episode usually consider the sleep sound and refreshing.

There is no connection between RBD and waking aggression. In fact, people with RBD are often described by their friends as being calm and friendly during the daytime.

RBD tends to start with minor symptoms (such as arm and leg movements and talking in one's sleep) that last for several years. Gradually, body movements become more pronounced, and episodes occur with increasing frequency.

RBD appears to be caused by a malfunction in a part of the brain stem that inhibits body movement. In experiments, cats with lesions of this site arch their backs, hiss, and bare their teeth during sleep. RBD frequently occurs in patients with neurological disorders such as narcolepsy, Parkinson's disease, and demen-

Case History

> When Jay, a sixty-six-year-old real estate lawyer, came to see me
> with his wife, he described an eight-year history of strange behavior
> during sleep. The episodes started after he was treated with Prozac
> for depression following prostate cancer surgery.
>
> Jay's wife related how he would typically wake her between 2
> and 3 A.M. by talking, shouting (at times using profanity), and
> laughing. He sometimes sat upright and moved his hands around,
> and on a few occasions, he actually struck his wife. The episodes
> were increasing in frequency and severity. There were times when
> he had gotten out bed and left the bedroom. Once, he went
> downstairs, walked into a table, fell down, and hit his head.
>
> If he woke up, Jay usually had some vague memory of his
> nighttime experiences. Sometimes he remembered feeling like he
> was being attacked or that people were coming into a room to get
> him. He also complained of daytime sleepiness, and his wife
> reported loud snoring and gasping for air at night.
>
> An overnight sleep study revealed that Jay had obstructive
> sleep apnea. Initially I suspected the partial awakenings from his

tia, as well as those who have had strokes. More than one-third
of people with RBD develop Parkinson's disease within three
years of the onset of the disorder, suggesting that similar brain
structures are implicated in both conditions. Antidepressant medications, particularly the selective serotonin reuptake inhibitors,
can bring on RBD.

RBD can almost always be treated successfully. The benzodiazepine clonazepam (Klonopin) reduces or eliminates the disorder
about 90 percent of the time. Other benzodiazepines may be similarly effective. Partners usually notice an improvement within the
first week, often beginning on the first night. If benzodiazepines
don't work, other medications, including dopamine stimulants
such as pramipexole (Mirapex) or anticonvulsants, may be tried.

OSA were triggering the unusual behavior. However, the strange occurrences continued at home even after he started using CPAP. He returned for a second sleep study, which showed that although the device was eliminating Jay's sleep apnea, he was frequently flailing his arms and legs while asleep. He also had one episode during REM sleep in which he punched his thigh while shouting.

The test results suggested that in addition to sleep apnea, Jay had both REM sleep behavior disorder and non-REM parasomnias (sleepwalking and sleeptalking). I prescribed the benzodiazepine temazepam (Restoril) to help him sleep more deeply and suppress his movements.

It took a little while to find the right dosage, but eventually Jay's disorders were brought under control. He still had occasional episodes, especially if he skipped his medicine or had a few drinks in the evening, but he slept better overall and felt more rested during the day. Jay's wife was much relieved, and she started sleeping better as well.

Until the problem is under control, and as a general precaution, it's advisable to make the room as safe as possible. Put sharp or breakable objects out of reach, and protect windows. Since there is a chance of Parkinson's disease developing, people with RBD should have an annual evaluation by a neurologist so the disease can be detected and treated as early as possible.

Nightmares

Sleep doctors define a nightmare as a dream so frightening that you wake up. (If you sleep through it, then it's just a bad dream.) Everybody has nightmares occasionally, and they generally are not cause for concern. Nightmares are especially common in children; we'll go over how parents should address kids' nightmares in Chapter 17.

Nightmares can be a problem if they occur so frequently that the person dreads going to sleep or gets so upset by the dreams that he or she has a hard time getting back to sleep. Both scenarios can cause sleep deprivation.

In these cases, identifying the source of the nightmares guides the treatment. For example, a traumatic event can lead to recurrent nightmares; seeing a mental health professional can help the individual deal with the emotional issues triggering the nightmares. Depression and schizophrenia are also associated with frequent nightmares.

Nightmares can be a side effect of medications, primarily those that affect neurotransmitter levels of the central nervous system, such as antidepressants, narcotics, and barbiturates (see Table 14.1). Nightmares also may occur when a person stops taking drugs that suppress REM sleep, such as benzodiazepines, causing a temporary increase in REM sleep. Talk to your doctor if you suspect medication is causing nightmares. Dream disturbances and nightmares also frequently accompany withdrawal from alcohol.

Other Parasomnias

Other parasomnias include sleeptalking, sleep-related eating disorder, bruxism, and bed-wetting (which is covered Chapter 17).

TABLE 14.1 Common Medications That Increase Frequency of Nightmares

Class	Medication
Antidepressant	Buproprion, paroxetine, fluoxetine
Antipsychotic	Thiothixene
Benzodiazepine	Triazolam, temazepam
Beta blocker	Metoprolol, propranolol, betaxolol, bisoprolol
Calcium channel blocker	Verapamil
Cholinesterase inhibitor	Donepezil
Nonsteroidal anti-inflammatory drugs (NSAIDs)	Naproxen

Talking in Your Sleep

Talking in one's sleep, or somniloquy, has no negative health consequences and is considered harmless. As a result, this phenomenon hasn't received much study. We do know that it's extremely common, and that like sleepwalking, it occurs most often during deep sleep. In these cases, people who talk in their sleep rarely remember what they said.

Less commonly, somniloquy occurs during REM sleep. In these instances, the spoken words may match the dream content. For example, the sleeper may call out "No, no!" and then report saying this in the dream as he or she witnessed something unpleasant. Sometimes the sleeper reports saying different words than those spoken.

Somniloquy can be disturbing to a partner's sleep. But tempting as it might be to put a pillow over the chatterer's head, the best thing is to let the episode play out. It's usually short-lived and the person returns to sleeping quietly. I recommend earplugs for sleeping partners if the problem happens regularly.

Sleep-Eating Disorders

There are two eating disorders associated with sleep, both of which are much more common in women than men.

- **Nocturnal eating syndrome.** This disorder is characterized by compulsive refrigerator raids during the night. People with this disorder are usually light sleepers who, upon awakening, feel that they won't be able to fall back to sleep unless they eat something. So they get out of bed, head to the refrigerator, and begin wolfing down food. The person is fully alert during the episode and can recall it the next day. This is more of an eating disorder than a sleep disorder, so it's usually best to seek treatment from a mental health professional who specializes in eating disorders. Since insomnia is a contributing factor, improving sleep hygiene often can help the individual's progress.

- **Sleep-related eating disorder.** This disorder is a variation of sleepwalking in which people get up and eat during a partial arousal from deep sleep. Often they consume unhealthy, high-calorie food that they would not eat during the daytime (such as cookie dough), which leads to weight gain. They may eat unappetizing food such as frozen pizzas, peanut butter on fish, or dog food. They are usually difficult to rouse during the episode, have no memory of it the next day, and are frequently sloppy or careless, which can result in injuries (such as burns or cuts from preparing food). The disorder does not seem to be prompted by hunger, since eating before bedtime often doesn't thwart it.

  A number of potential triggers have been identified: medications such as the mood stabilizer lithium and the benzodiazepine receptor agonist zolpidem (Ambien); psychological problems such as bulimia and mood and personality disorders; and other sleep disorders, particularly insomnia but also sleep apnea, narcolepsy, and PLMD.

  Sleep eaters often have a history of sleepwalking, so this phenomenon is considered more of a sleep disorder than an eating disorder. Eliminating sleepwalking will stop the trips to the refrigerator. Treatment with medication is often effective. Dopamine agents, anticonvulsants, antidepressants, and opiates are among the drugs prescribed.

Bruxism

Bruxism, or teeth grinding, occurs when people clench their top and bottom teeth together, especially the back teeth. The stressful force of clenching causes pressure on the muscles, tissues, and other structures around the jaw. This can wear down tooth enamel and lead to fractured fillings, injured gums, jaw pain and soreness (also known as temporomandibular joint dysfunction), headaches, earaches, and facial pain. In addition, bruxism causes a surprisingly loud and disturbing sound—imagine rocks being ground together—that can wake up one's partner.

Unlike most parasomnias, which occur either during deep sleep or REM sleep, bruxism occurs mostly during the lighter stages of sleep (Stages 1 and 2). The cause isn't known—possible triggers include stress and anxiety; the shape of the jaw; caffeine, nicotine, and alcohol; and medication.

An estimated 8 percent of people grind their teeth during sleep, usually without being aware of it. Some do it during the daytime as well, most often during situations that make them feel tense or anxious.

Bruxism sometimes goes away without treatment, especially when it occurs in children. When it persists and is severe enough to warrant treatment, a number of therapies can be effective, although there's often some trial and error involved in finding one that works.

If bruxism is caused by a dental problem, it may stop when the teeth are repaired and realigned. For some people, wearing a nocturnal bite plate or splint takes care of the problem. Others benefit from stress-reduction therapies and cutting down on their intake of alcohol and caffeine. Pharmacologic therapies include prescription muscle relaxants, antidepressants, and dopamine agents. However, scientific studies to determine the best regimen are still needed. In severe cases in which patients haven't responded to other treatments, some doctors now use botulinum toxin (Botox) injections.

CHAPTER 15

Disturbances of Sleep Timing: DSP and ASP

As you know, the circadian rhythm of sleep and wakefulness strongly influences when you're sleepiest and most alert. Ideally, your sleep/wake rhythm is synchronized with your lifestyle. In other words, if you naturally start to feel sleepy around 10:30 P.M., then you're in a good position to fall asleep at 11:00 and get up at about 7:30 A.M., which works out well for people who keep traditional daytime hours.

If your schedule strays from the sleep/wake pattern set by your circadian rhythm, you may have trouble sleeping when you need to. People with circadian timing disorders have extreme cases of this problem. With delayed sleep phase disorder (DSP), the circadian rhythm is delayed by several hours, so drowsiness doesn't arrive until the middle of the night. With advanced sleep phase disorder (ASP), the circadian rhythm advances by several hours, so sleepiness arrives very early in the evening. Let's look further at the timing issues underlying these disorders and how they're treated.

Symptoms of Delayed and Advanced Sleep Phase Disorders

People with DSP are natural night owls who, left to their own devices, stay up late, often not falling asleep until 2, 3, or even 4 A.M. Then they sleep until the late morning or early afternoon. If your job entails working the evening shift and you can sleep in afterward, this isn't a drawback—in fact, it's ideal. But if you need to be at work by 9 A.M., then it's a problem.

People with DSP have great difficulty falling asleep at a traditional bedtime. At an hour when most people start to yawn, they're near peak alertness. If they try to sleep at 11 P.M., they experience what seems like ordinary insomnia—they toss and turn for hours and then finally fall asleep.

However, unlike some insomniacs, people with DSP have no trouble staying asleep. The problem is that they have a hard time getting out of bed on time in the morning, since the morning alarm curtails what would have been a lengthy sleep block. This leaves them sleep deprived, which leads to excessive daytime sleepiness that can cause serious problems at work, at the wheel, in marital relationships, and so on. People with DSP often compensate for lost sleep during the workweek by sleeping additional hours on the weekend; ten- or even twelve-hour blocks lasting until midafternoon are not uncommon.

DSP is most common in adolescence, with a prevalence as high as 7 percent, but most teens outgrow it by young adulthood. An estimated 0.7 percent of adults have the disorder, and about 10 percent of people who go to a sleep clinic with a complaint of insomnia are diagnosed with DSP.

DSP's precise cause isn't known, but it's clearly a circadian rhythm problem. You may recall from Chapter 2 that the light/dark cycle, as well as time cues such as clocks, keeps the circadian rhythm on a 24-hour schedule for most people. However, if these zeitgebers are removed—say, if a person lives underground in unchanging dim light without clocks or other time cues—the cir-

Free-Running Circadian Rhythms

Most totally blind people have "free-running" circadian rhythms. Their bodies do not respond to cycles of light and darkness, enabling circadian rhythms to run in cycles greater than twenty-four hours. The disorder, formally known as non-twenty-four-hour sleep-wake syndrome, pushes people toward a progressively later bedtime and a different sleep block each day, which frequently causes insomnia and daytime sleepiness. In rare instances, sighted individuals have free-running circadian rhythms. For both blind and sighted sufferers, the disorder can often be treated with timed doses of melatonin.

cadian rhythm usually runs on a slightly longer schedule, about 24.2 hours.

Experiments in these conditions have found that the natural circadian rhythm varies by individual, from as short as 23 hours to as long as 25.5, with the majority falling between 24.1 and 24.5 hours. In these experiments, most people go to bed progressively later each night—usually by thirty to sixty minutes—so that after two weeks, they are unwittingly sleeping in the daytime and staying awake at night.

For most people, this tendency for the circadian rhythm to run a bit more than twenty-four hours isn't a problem in real life. The zeitgebers do a good job of pulling them back to a twenty-four-hour cycle. This isn't the case for people with DSP; their lengthened cycle constantly pushes them toward a later bedtime. This may result from a decreased sensitivity to light and darkness or from some other cause. Part of the problem is behavioral—people choose to stay up late for social reasons, which increases their exposure to artificial light and shifts their circadian rhythm. But studies have shown that most people with DSP have changes in their circadian rhythm regardless of behavior.

Case History

When Alex, a twenty-six-year-old teacher, made an appointment to see me at the clinic, he insisted that we meet in the afternoon—morning was not an option. He explained that, for several years, he had had trouble getting up in the morning. No matter how much he slept, he couldn't get up on time. He had two alarms in his room but repeatedly slept through them. When he did finally get up, it took him a couple of hours to get going. His head felt like it was in a fog, not clearing until midmorning. He drank two cups of coffee to help him get through.

To get to school on time, he had to get up at 6 A.M. He tried to get enough sleep by going to bed by 9:30 P.M. but had a hard time falling asleep, taking one to two hours to drift off. Once asleep, he slept straight through until morning. On weekends he slept until noon. He would just start feeling better on Sunday when the trouble would start all over again.

In college, Alex stayed up late and slept late and had no sleep problems. His difficulties began when he started working. Summer

People with ASP have the opposite problem as those with DSP—their circàdian rhythm is shifted so that their sleep block starts earlier and ends earlier than most people's, leading to an earlier-than-normal bedtime. People with ASP may start to get sleepy around 8 P.M. and nod off shortly thereafter. Then they wake up between 3 and 5 A.M.

Again, if allowed to follow their own schedule, those with ASP have no trouble falling asleep, have normal sleep architecture, and are not sleepy during waking hours. Even so, people with this condition often perceive that they have insomnia—the type in which you wake up early in the morning—and will list insomnia as their major complaint when they go to a sleep clinic. While it's usually not difficult for people with ASP to hold down daytime jobs, they often have impaired social lives, since they're

vacation, when he could follow his old college schedule, was the only time he felt well rested. Alex had no other medical problems or symptoms of other sleep disorders and was not taking any medications.

Based on his description, it was clear that Alex had delayed sleep phase disorder. To shift his circadian rhythm to an earlier schedule, we had him start using a bright light box when he got up in the morning. He also took 3 milligrams of melatonin at night shortly before his desired sleep time. For the first week, he took a short-acting benzodiazepine receptor agonist, Ambien, to help him get to sleep while shifting his schedule.

Alex did quite well and was able to get to work on time as long as he kept to a strict schedule and used his light box in the morning. Come summer vacation, he would let himself go back to his old schedule. Then each fall he would shift his schedule again in time for the start of school.

reluctant to participate in evening activities for fear of falling asleep.

The cause of ASP isn't known; it may result from having a circadian rhythm that runs in a cycle of less than twenty-four hours. The disorder is less common than DSP, and it occurs most commonly among older people. Some tendency toward being more of a morning person is natural with age, but with ASP, the problem is more severe.

Treatments for DSP and ASP

Treatment for DSP and ASP is only necessary if the person wants or needs to be on a more traditional sleep/wake schedule. Treatment options include chronotherapy, bright light, and melatonin.

Chronotherapy

Chronotherapy means deliberately changing one's bedtime and wake-up time to shift the circadian rhythm. For DSP, chronotherapy entails successively delaying bedtime by three hours per day, until the desired bedtime is reached. Then the person must rigidly adhere to the new sleep/wake schedule.

Let's look at an example of someone who falls asleep at 2 A.M. but wants to fall asleep at 11 P.M. During chronotherapy, his or her bedtime would move to 5 A.M. on Sunday, 8 A.M. on Monday, 11 A.M. on Tuesday, 2 P.M. on Wednesday, 5 P.M. on Thursday, 8 P.M. on Friday, and 11 P.M. on Saturday. From there, he or she would try to stick to going to bed at 11 P.M. and rising at 7 A.M. As you can see, this requires having a week that can be devoted to therapy, since you could not keep to a normal routine while rotating your sleep block around the clock.

Maintaining a consistent wake-up time once the desired bedtime is reached is crucial, since sleeping past it will only make it hard to fall asleep the next night. People who deviate from the new schedule quickly revert to their old sleep/wake schedule, requiring them to go through the whole process again. To prevent this from occurring, sleep medication is sometimes used during the shift or immediately afterward to help cement the new bedtime.

Chronotherapy for DSP can be effective, provided the individual does not face pressure from outside sources that interfere with the ability to maintain the unusual hours required by the treatment. For example, it may not be feasible for people with full-time jobs or parents with young children.

Although it's possible to use chronotherapy for ASP—advancing the bedtime by three hours per night (from 9 P.M. to 6 P.M. to 3 P.M. and so on) until the desired bedtime is reached and then maintaining the new schedule, it's much harder to do and is rarely recommended.

Bright Light

This treatment grew out of the discovery that exposure to bright light within a few hours of the body's low point in body temper-

FIGURE 15.1 Light Therapy for Sleep Phase Disorders

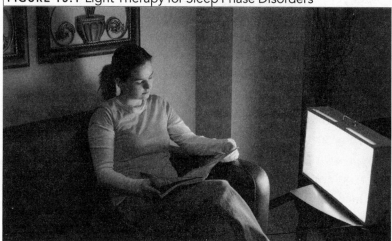

Patients with circadian rhythm disorders can use bright light therapy to shift their sleep/wake rhythm. Individuals typically sit near the light source for thirty minutes to an hour.   Copyright © Scientifica/Visuals Unlimited

ature—which occurs during the overnight hours—shifts the circadian rhythm. A dose of bright light after the temperature minimum advances the circadian rhythm, while a dose before it delays the rhythm.

One way to think of light therapy is that you are using light to trick the circadian clock in your brain into thinking that the outside environment has changed. The clock senses artificial evening light as a delay in sunset and shifts the sleep/wake cycle to accommodate this new environment. If artificial bright light occurs early in the morning, it's perceived as an earlier sunrise and the sleep block advances. You're using light to tap into the same mechanism that allows your body to accommodate normally to the change from standard to daylight savings time.

Regardless of which direction we want the shift to go, the person sits near a commercially manufactured light box that uses fluorescent bulbs for thirty minutes to an hour (see Figure 15.1). It's OK to keep one's eyes open, but it isn't necessary (or advisable) to look directly at the light—relaxed activities such as reading, writing, or eating are recommended.

For people with DSP, light is usually administered immediately upon waking in the morning (between 7 and 9 A.M.). This advances the circadian rhythm, so the next night it should be easier for the person to go to sleep an hour or so earlier. Evening light can undo the phase advance, so avoidance of bright indoor or outdoor lights is necessary to maintain the effect.

For people with ASP, the timing is reversed. Patients sit by the light box in the early evening (between 7 and 9 P.M.), which delays the circadian rhythm. It's helpful to avoid morning sunlight that would negate the treatment's effects.

Once the desired bedtime is reached, some people can discontinue bright light therapy. But most need to continue with daily exposure to help them stay on the new sleep/wake schedule

No prescription is needed for light therapy, and light boxes can be purchased for $300 to $500. However, since there are many variables—how much light, at what time, and for how long—the initial treatment should ideally be monitored closely by a doctor with expertise in circadian physiology. If light therapy isn't working, you may be delivering the light at the wrong time, and it's difficult to detect where you are in your circadian cycle outside of a laboratory. Side effects are uncommon but may include headaches, nausea, and eye irritation. In rare cases, bright light treatment can trigger a manic state characterized by restlessness, irritability, and insomnia.

Most studies on this therapy have used white light from a light box. Two newer methods of delivering light—light visors and dawn simulators—also are available. Light visors are portable devices shaped like sun visors that deliver lower levels of light directly to the eye. Dawn simulators are devices that you plug into a bedroom lamp so the light level in your room rises gradually, simulating sunrise at a time you choose. These devices have not been as extensively tested as light boxes, but they may change your circadian rhythm just as effectively.

Most recently, several studies have found that blue light shifts the circadian rhythm more effectively than white. Researchers are now investigating whether low doses of blue light might be as effective as (and less obtrusive than) higher doses of white light.

Melatonin

In lab studies, doses of synthetic melatonin have been shown to shift the circadian rhythm in the opposite direction from the shift with bright light, leading sleep doctors to believe that it too can play a role in treating sleep timing disorders. As with bright light, proper timing of the dosage is vital or the person's problem can be worsened.

People with DSP may benefit from melatonin several hours before bedtime (which advances the circadian rhythm), and people with ASP may be helped by a dose in the morning (which delays the circadian rhythm). The usual dose is 3 to 5 milligrams. Unfortunately, since melatonin sold in stores is not regulated by the FDA, there is no guarantee that the product you buy will have the correct dose.

Ramelteon (Rozerem), a new sleep medication that stimulates the same receptors in the brain that melatonin does and shifts the circadian rhythm, may be helpful in treating timing disorders. More research is needed, but it's likely this drug will become an option for treating DSP and ASP.

Sleeping Pills

Standard sleep medication can also have a role in treating timing disorders. When someone has difficulty adapting to a new schedule, a short course of medication may be helpful to stabilize a new circadian rhythm when combined with chronotherapy or light therapy. This should only be done under the direction of your doctor.

CHAPTER 16

Challenging Sleep Situations: Jet Lag, Shift Work, and Drowsy Driving

In a perfect world—or at least a sleep doctor's perfect world— you'd go to bed and wake up at the same time every day. The human body craves regularity, so sticking to the same daily schedule keeps your circadian system running smoothly and increases your likelihood of falling and staying asleep.

Of course, reality has a way of throwing us off a twenty-four-hour routine, which in turn can cause sleep problems and other health complaints. In this chapter, we'll look at two common situations in which the circadian rhythm gets out of whack—jet lag and shift work—and how you can best minimize the problems they cause. We'll also cover another vital sleep-related challenge: how to stay awake at the wheel.

Jet Lag

Just about everyone who travels experiences jet lag. It can be a minor inconvenience or a major shock to your system, depending on the circumstances. Common symptoms include daytime sleepiness, insomnia, frequent nighttime awakenings, headaches, difficulty concentrating, impaired judgment, and upset stomach.

Jet lag's cause is fairly simple. The short version is that flying forces you to cross time zones faster than your body can adapt to the change. But why is this so? As we've seen, your circadian rhythm of sleep and wakefulness normally runs on a cycle of approximately twenty-four hours, with the daily cycle of light and darkness and other time cues keeping it from drifting off schedule. Rapid crossing of time zones gives you a shortened or lengthened day, plus a new light/dark schedule at your destination. This puts your internal sleep/wake rhythm out of sync with the external environment.

The sleep/wake rhythm *can* adjust to the new time zone, but it takes its sweet time, generally moving approximately an hour or two a day. That means, for example, that when you fly from New York to London, crossing five time zones, the local time may be 7 A.M., but your body's biological clock still thinks it's 2 A.M. Your brain gets conflicting signals from this five-hour time shift—the morning sunlight says wake up, but your internal clock and the many hours you've gone without sleep say go to bed.

While your circadian rhythm makes the gradual transition from the old light/dark schedule to the new one, you're liable to have trouble falling asleep. Once awake, your internal clock may tell you it's time for bed, making it difficult to stay awake. Making matters worse, travel itself is often stressful and exhausting—staying up late packing and getting ready for the trip; making the airport commute; and dealing with security, luggage, flight delays, crowded planes, and so forth.

Jet lag's severity depends on several factors:

- **Direction of travel.** In general, it's easier to fly westward, since that extends the day. As we saw in the last chapter, circadian rhythms have a tendency to run on cycles of slightly more than twenty-four hours, so it's easier to adapt to a longer-than-usual day than a shorter one.

- **Distance.** The more time zones you cross, the longer it takes to get accustomed to the light/dark cycle of your destination. With time shifts greater than six hours, different circadian rhythms (sleep/wake, body temperature, hormone secretion) may shift in opposite directions, further prolonging jet lag symptoms.
- **Individual circadian flexibility.** Some people's circadian rhythms are more flexible than others, enabling them to adapt more quickly to time zone changes. In general, older people are more susceptible to jet lag, because the circadian system becomes less adaptable with age.

Minimizing the Pain: The Basics

Once your destination is set, there's not much you can do about the general factors. But there are steps you can take to minimize jet lag. Here are some commonly used strategies:

- **Don't time-shift on short trips.** If your return flight is within a day or two of your arrival, you may fare best by staying on your "home" sleep/wake schedule. Keep your watch set to the home time; go to bed, wake up, and eat meals at your usual home times; and avoid sunlight as much as possible (because it pushes your circadian rhythms to the "away" time). If you're on a business trip, schedule appointments for times when you would be alert at home. You may feel out of place with this strategy—since you'll be going to bed and waking up at unconventional local times— but it really works on quick trips.
- **Start switching before you arrive.** For trips lasting longer than a day or two, you'll want to make the switch to the new time zone. One way to make the adjustment more quickly is to get a jump on things before you leave. For a day or two before your flight, move your mealtimes and bedtime closer to the schedule of your destination. For example, if you are flying east to west, progressively stay up one hour later and sleep in one hour later for the two days

prior to leaving. Change your watch to the destination time zone when you board (or earlier), and try to sleep on the plane if you're in the air during your destination's nighttime.

- **Upon arrival, switch as rapidly as possible.** Once you land, avoid the temptation to go to bed at what would have been your usual time. Try to eat meals, go to bed, and wake up on the schedule of the new time zone, even if this means forcing yourself to stay awake additional hours or getting up at what feels like an ungodly hour.

- **Take a short, strategic nap.** If you find yourself completely exhausted during the daytime, take a twenty- to thirty-minute afternoon nap. This should boost your alertness and help you stay awake until your new bedtime. However—and this is important—avoid longer naps and naps of any duration in the evening. Both will make it harder to fall asleep at night, prolonging jet lag.

- **Use the sun to your advantage.** Remember, light has the most potent effect on resetting the circadian clock. For the first day or two of your trip, spend as much time outdoors as possible to let daylight reset your internal clock. If you need to wake up earlier in the new setting (flying west to east), get out in the early-morning sun. If you need to wake up later (flying east to west), expose yourself to late-afternoon sunlight.

- **Watch what you drink.** Drink plenty of water to avoid dehydration. Avoid caffeine and alcohol, which can worsen the physical symptoms of jet lag and disturb sleep.

- **Practice good sleep hygiene.** Good habits for sleeping under normal circumstances take on extra significance when you're jet-lagged, since you're trying to sleep at times when you're body isn't 100 percent geared for it. Use window shades to make it as dark as possible and wear earplugs to block out sound. Avoid heavy, spicy meals, which you're likely to have a hard time digesting. A good daytime workout—such as a jog, a long brisk walk, or laps in a hotel pool—can also make a difference.

Additional Measures

The preceding tactics make jet lag tolerable for most people. However, if you try them and still find that jet lag knocks you for a loop, you may wish to consider other measures, such as prescription sleep medications and melatonin.

Sleep Medication. Sleeping pills won't help your body adapt to the new time zone. They can even prolong jet lag, if you end up sleeping far past your destination's traditional wake-up time. That being said, sleep medication, such as one of the shorter-lasting benzodiazepine receptor agonists, can help with short-term insomnia during the first few nights of a trip, especially if your new bedtime falls during your circadian time for alertness. Sleeping pills also can be helpful if you want to sleep during a long flight in which you're in the air while it's nighttime at your destination. Your doctor can help you decide if the benefits outweigh the drawbacks.

Synthetic Melatonin. Since the 1990s, researchers have studied whether synthetic melatonin's proven ability to shift circadian rhythms can alleviate jet lag. The studies have led to conflicting results, but the general consensus is that the following approach, developed by Josephine Arendt and Stephen Deacon at the University of Surrey in the United Kingdom, can reduce insomnia, daytime fatigue, and other jet lag symptoms:

- If you're traveling eastward, take one 3- to 5-milligram capsule on departure day (if necessary, on the flight) between 6 and 7 P.M. on your home time. After arrival, take a capsule at the local bedtime (around 11 P.M.) for up to four days.
- If you're traveling westward, don't take any melatonin before your flight. After arrival, take one capsule at the local bedtime for up to four days.

Even though it's available over the counter, it's a good idea to consult your doctor if you're considering taking melatonin for the

The Wide World of Shift Work Schedules

A surefire conversation starter with someone who works at a twenty-four-hour company is to ask what schedule the person works and how he or she feels about it. Unless you've worked nights yourself, you probably haven't thought about the many variables:

- **Eight-hour versus twelve-hour.** A few shift workers work ten-hour shifts, but most work eights or twelves, since those lengths divide evenly into the twenty-four-hour operation many employers require. Many shift workers prefer twelve-hour schedules because they provide more days off. However, longer shifts can lead to sleep deprivation that interferes with work performance.
- **Fixed versus rotating.** On a fixed schedule, an individual always works the same shift. On a rotating shift, a person switches from nights to days (on twelves) or works a combination of days, evenings, and nights (on eights).
- **Speed of rotation.** Some rotating schedules rotate slowly, meaning people work the same shift two weeks or more before moving to a new one. On a fast rotation, people move to a different shift whenever they return from days off. Some schedules, including many in Europe, rotate even faster,

first time, to review potential health concerns and make sure you time the dose properly. Melatonin can cause drowsiness, so make sure you don't need to be alert (that is, driving or operating heavy machinery) when you first take it.

Shift Work

More than 20 percent of workers in the industrialized world regularly work at night. That includes large numbers of people in twenty-four-hour industries such as power, mining, transportation, manufacturing, health care, and emergency services (police,

meaning a person might work one or two consecutive days, evenings, and nights *between* days off. Faster schedules don't allow time for shifting the circadian cycle, so workers have the fewest number of days sleeping at odds with their circadian rhythm.

- **Direction of rotation.** Rotating eight-hour schedules can go either forward (days to evenings to nights) or backward (days to nights to evenings). Because of the slightly longer than twenty-four-hour length of the circadian cycle, forward-rotating schedules are theoretically easier to adapt to than backward-rotating schedules.
- **Shift change time.** The morning shift change usually occurs sometime between 6 and 8 A.M. An early changeover can make it easier for people on the night shift to fall asleep when they get home but may lead those on the day shift to become sleep deprived, since they need to rise so early.

There is no consensus on what constitutes the best shift work schedule, since people have different priorities based on their social lives and physiological needs. In general, people tend to like their schedule more if they have a say in choosing it.

firefighters, EMTs, and so on). Dozens of shift work schedules exist. Whatever the specifics, schedules that require work through the overnight hours are the most difficult physically.

Like jet lag, shift work is challenging because it forces you to live out of sync with the natural sleep/wake rhythm. Shift workers need to be alert at times when their bodies are naturally drawn to sleep, and they must try to sleep at times when their bodies are geared for wakefulness.

Compared to air travelers, shift workers have one key disadvantage—their circadian rhythms never fully adapt to their new "time zone" (being awake at night and sleeping during the daytime). One reason is that whereas the light/dark cycle at a traveler's destination helps the body get oriented to the new time zone, the light/dark cycle for a shift worker remains in opposition to his or her sleep/wake schedule. No matter how many days, months, or years a person works at night, the morning sunlight that greets him or her when the night shift ends perpetually sends a message to the brain that it's time to wake up, not go to sleep.

Another factor working against permanent circadian adaptation to the night shift is that people tend to revert to a traditional sleep/wake schedule on their days off, so they can spend leisure time with family and friends. When this happens, the partial adaptation to night work that may occur from working successive night shifts is lost. When it's time to go back to work, the individual's body is once again fully oriented for a traditional sleep/wake schedule.

The bottom line is that most shift workers live in a state of constant circadian disruption. (The exception would be someone who works exclusively on night shifts and who also stays awake at night and sleeps during the daytime on days off—a rare occurrence.) This disruption has a direct effect on sleep, with shift workers typically averaging just four to six hours of sleep per twenty-four hours. Often, sleep is severely fragmented—after coming off a night shift, a person may sleep for three or four hours but then repeatedly wake up over the next few hours. This results in chronic sleep deprivation, which often leads to difficulty staying awake on the job and at the wheel, causing industrial and auto accidents.

Research has linked shift work to a number of health problems, with the strongest evidence pertaining to the heart and stomach. For example, long-term shift work increases the risk of heart disease by up to 30 to 40 percent, and it may also contribute to hypertension. Shift workers are more likely to have both minor gastrointestinal (GI) problems (constipation, diarrhea, excessive gas, and heartburn) as well as serious long-term GI ailments (chronic gastritis and peptic ulcers).

Case History

Shift work is a necessity at a sleep lab. Sleep studies must be performed when most people sleep—at night—and trained technologists are needed to run the tests and work with patients. Since shift work is inevitable, we do everything we can at our clinic to create the best possible environment for our shift workers.

The first step is education. During our techs' training, before they ever work at night, they're instructed on the basics of sleep and circadian rhythms. Next, we review ways to cope with shift work—all the strategies described in this chapter. They then spend some time observing on the night shift to make sure they can tolerate it.

Once on the job, we also try to provide an optimal environment. The techs are encouraged to work as a team, covering for each other to make sure details are not missed. The lab includes a refreshment area with free coffee, tea, and hot chocolate. Light boxes are available to use during the night to increase alertness. On breaks, they are encouraged to take naps. One big advantage of working in a sleep lab is that at the end of their shift, after the patients have gone, the techs can nap in one of the beds if they're too drowsy to drive.

Finally, if they are still having trouble coping with night work, they are encouraged to consult with a sleep specialist—us! We provide access to our sleep specialists as a type of occupational health program.

Many researchers also believe that shift work can cause or contribute to mental health problems (such as mood swings, irritability, and mild depression), and that if a person is predisposed to a more severe problem such as manic depression, shift work can serve as a trigger that brings on the disorder. Shift work may pose reproductive risks, increasing the likelihood of delays in conception, premature delivery, and miscarriage. Working at night can also take a heavy social toll, increasing the likelihood of divorce and making it hard for parents to spend time with their children and for single people to have satisfying social lives.

Shift work tends to get harder with age, since it becomes harder to stay asleep in the daytime as you age. It's common for shift workers who coped reasonably well with shiftwork in their twenties and thirties to start struggling in their forties and fifties.

Although working shifts is generally more difficult than working a nine-to-five job, it's worth pointing out that not everyone has a hard time with it. In fact, some people actually prefer it to daytime work. These people are often night owls who have no trouble staying awake at night and sleeping during the daytime. For such people, having to be at work at 8 A.M. would be the true hardship. The higher salaries and increased independence also make shift work attractive to some people.

Coping Strategies

The following techniques can help you cope with the challenges of shift work.

- **Recognize the importance of sleep and make it a priority.** This holds true for everyone, but it's especially critical for shift workers.
- **Create a haven for sleep.** Sleeping in the daytime is a supreme challenge. Along with the circadian aspect of trying to sleep when the body is geared for wakefulness, you have to contend with sunlight and noise from phone calls, lawn mowers, children playing, and so on. Some shift workers construct special sound- and lightproof sleeping quarters in an isolated room of the house. If this isn't possible, at least make your bedroom as quiet and dark as possible, with tightly sealed windows and blackout curtains or shades.
- **Protect your sleep.** Make sure family and friends know not to bother you unless it's an emergency. Buy a VCR or digital recorder so you don't skip sleep for TV, and use an

answering machine with a ringer (and outgoing message) that you can turn off while you sleep. Just as a nine-to-fiver wouldn't schedule the electrician to come in the middle of the night, you should schedule appointments in the late afternoon—after your primary sleep block.

- **Develop a sleep strategy.** While circadian disruption is inevitable, shift workers should take steps to minimize the jolt to the body as much as possible. Every schedule has different features, so you need to put some thought into what's going to work best. Whatever plan you develop, stick to it. If you're new to a particular schedule, map out when you plan to sleep. You might also seek out some veterans at your company to ask what works for them.

  If you work night shifts from Monday to Friday and have weekends off, consider staying on your work schedule over the weekend. If this isn't feasible, try to avoid going all the way back to a daytime schedule on Saturday and Sunday. Staying up late and sleeping late on days off will ease your transition to and from workdays.

  If you have more than a couple of days off between night shifts, then you'll probably choose to resume a standard sleep schedule on your days off. Again, the key is making a smooth transition. Staying up late and sleeping late for a night or two before your first night of work should make the first couple of night shifts easier.

  Some schedules lend themselves to a concept known as anchor sleep. The idea here is that you can minimize circadian disruption by always sleeping during the same three- or four-hour block, whether it's a workday or a day off. For example, if you sleep from 8 A.M. to 2 P.M. (or later) on workdays and 3 A.M. to 11 A.M. on off days, then the block from 8 A.M. to 11 A.M. serves as anchor sleep.

- **Allow for recovery days.** Whatever your work schedule, it's wise to designate the first day after your last night shift as a recovery day, during which you catch up on lost sleep and take care of local errands and odds and ends at home. Try to schedule more strenuous activities (trips, sports, and the like) for subsequent days off.

- **Use strategic naps.** Shift workers, being chronically sleep deprived, stand to benefit from naps that supplement their longest sleep block. Rather than napping randomly, it's preferable to make naps a part of your overall sleep strategy. The best results have come from nap breaks at work; research shows that a midshift nap increases alertness and decreases sleepiness and circadian disruption. Unfortunately, most workplaces don't permit on-site napping, so supplementary daytime naps are often the only option. Someone who has trouble staying asleep after a night shift might plan on sleeping from 8 A.M. to noon, supplemented by a two- or three-hour nap sometime before returning to work. Those who can sleep longer in the morning may still want to squeeze in a short nap before work.

- **Avoid morning sunlight.** If you choose to sleep in the morning following night shifts, try to get home and into bed as quickly as possible. To minimize exposure to sunlight, wear sunglasses on your drive home and don't stop to shop or get gas. The more sunlight you're exposed to, the more likely you are to have trouble falling and staying asleep.

- **Guard against alertness lapses.** The overnight hours are high-risk times for accidents, with the predawn hours typically the toughest. Learn to recognize the signs of fatigue (such as concentration problems, difficulty in keeping your eyes open, and an inability to remember the last five minutes), and then take action. As noted earlier, the best response is to take a break and a short nap, if your employer permits this; a nap can refresh you enough to get through the shift. Other common strategies include standing, stretching, or walking around; talking to coworkers; and having a snack. Keeping the work environment well lit also helps, since bright light has an energizing effect. A fifteen-to twenty-minute break in front of a bright light box can ward off fatigue for an hour or two.

- **Use caffeine wisely.** Caffeine boosts alertness, but excessive consumption can make it hard to sleep after a night shift. You'll get the best bang for your buck if you limit yourself to one or two caffeinated beverages per shift, at times when you need it most. Nursing your cup may be helpful—recent research suggests that frequent but small amounts of caffeine can maintain an increased level of alertness at work without making it harder to sleep when you get home. You might also establish a caffeine cutoff time, after which you switch to juice or water.

- **Use medications judiciously.** I don't usually recommend sleeping pills for shift workers. Unlike jet lag, shift work is not a temporary phenomenon. So once a shift worker starts using sleep medication, there's a tendency to rely on it all the time, which may pose long-term health risks and can lead to tolerance and dependence. However, I recognize that many shift workers do use sleep aids. If you go this route, avoid over-the-counter drugs—prescription medications work better and have fewer side effects—and be sure to follow your doctor's instructions.

Once you've worked the same schedule for a while, you'll probably notice that sleep is worse some days than others and that you can reliably predict those days. For instance, some shift workers find it's hardest to sleep after the first shift of the week, because they've been on a regular schedule on their days off. Later in the week, they're so tired it's easier to sleep. In this case, it might help to use sleeping medication for the first day or two of the week to minimize this predictable sleep disruption.

Recently, researchers showed that the stimulant modafinil (Provigil) significantly reduced sleepiness during shift work, with a slight improvement in job performance as well. The drug did not return alertness or performance to daytime levels, but the study volunteers fared better with modafinil than with a placebo.

While stimulants such as modafinil can be a useful tool to promote alertness, they do not change the circadian factors causing sleepiness and do not eliminate the need for sleep. Medication, whether stimulants or sedatives, should only be used after consultation with your doctor.

- **If necessary, have an exit strategy.** People who make a commitment to getting enough sleep stand a good chance of tolerating the night shift. However, some people—through no fault of their own—just aren't cut out for shift work. Usually this stems from an innate inability to sleep more than a few hours during the daylight hours. If you frequently fall asleep on the job due to chronic sleep deprivation and experience other health ailments as a result of your work schedule (significant weight gain, GI distress, mood swings, and so on), consider employment alternatives that don't require you to be on the job at 4 A.M.

Drowsy Driving

The National Highway Traffic Safety Administration conservatively estimates that one hundred thousand car crashes in the United States each year are the direct result of driver fatigue, causing more than fifteen hundred deaths and seventy-one thousand injuries. A 2005 Canadian survey found that one in five drivers admitted they had nodded off or fallen asleep at the wheel at least once in the previous year. A 2006 review by the Institutes of Medicine of the National Academy of Sciences found that almost 20 percent of all serious car accidents and 57 percent of fatal accidents are associated with driver sleepiness. Certain groups face an elevated risk of drowsy driving accidents—including people under twenty-six, shift workers, commercial drivers, and people with undiagnosed sleep disorders such as sleep apnea—but they can happen to anyone.

Studies show that sleep deprivation has the same impact on your ability to drive as drinking alcohol does. People who have been without sleep for twenty-four hours perform as badly on driving and other performance tests as people with blood alcohol levels of 0.10, which is above the legal limit in every state. The combination of sleep deprivation and alcohol is even worse.

How can you reduce your accident risk? Let's look at the options, from most effective to least effective. You won't be surprised to learn that getting enough sleep is by far the most effective thing you can do to avoid attention lapses on the road. People who get sufficient sleep (seven and a half or eight hours for most people) and stay off the road after they've been awake for more than fifteen hours rarely nod off at the wheel.

Timing your drive wisely also improves your chances of staying alert. Due to circadian factors, driving late at night or in the early morning increases your chances of falling asleep. Although more accidents happen during the day because more cars are on the road, predawn accidents are more likely to be fatal, since people often fall asleep and drive off the road at high speeds.

If you find your head bobbing while you're driving on a long trip, that's a sure sign that you need some sleep. Get off the road, and if possible check into a hotel for the night and resume driving in the morning.

If waiting until the next day to complete your journey is not an option, find a safe place where you can take a nap. Unlike most other measures, a nap gets to the heart of the problem—you're sleep deprived, and a nap provides sleep. Once you wake up, allow yourself ten or fifteen minutes to shake any grogginess that may linger.

While caffeine is not a substitute for sleep, it does boost alertness. You're best off using it sparingly, since caffeine's effect diminishes at high doses. In other words, your first and second cup of coffee will provide a significant lift, but your fourth and fifth provide little or no benefit (in addition to making it hard to sleep later and irritating your stomach). One strategy is to pull off the road, drink one or two cups of coffee or tea, and then take a short nap. By the time you're up and ready to drive, the caffeine will have kicked in and you'll have the double effect of sleep and caffeine to help you stay alert.

Compared to sleep, napping, and caffeine, other measures are relatively ineffective. Despite your best intentions, you can and will fall asleep at the wheel. Willpower is not a factor; like a car that's out of gas, the brain automatically shuts down at a certain level of sleep deprivation.

Driving with passengers theoretically can help, since having someone to talk with keeps the driver's mind engaged, and the passenger can monitor the driver's behavior. However, it's not a surefire solution because passengers often fall asleep, leaving the driver to fight sleep alone.

Many people believe pulling the car over and stretching or doing exercise for five or ten minutes is a smart thing to do when they're tired. Unfortunately, research hasn't shown this to be an effective way to avoid nodding off. The problem is that, at best, exercise and stretching provide only a temporary boost of alertness. Once a driver gets back on the road, he or she is back to the previous low alertness level within a few minutes.

Other popular measures are even less effective. Putting the air conditioner on full blast, sitting in an awkward position, and playing annoying music have minimal benefit and shouldn't be relied on. Slapping oneself in the face and chewing on ice may keep a person awake for the duration of the activity, but the small benefit ends once the activity is over. Ordinary activities such as singing along with the radio, taking off one's shoes, and opening the window provide little or no benefit. In fact, they may actually be counterproductive because they can give a sleepy driver a false sense of security.

Drowsy driving is more than just an inconvenience—it is life-threatening. Drowsy driving accidents often involve other cars and pedestrians, so you're not just gambling with your own life.

The public and policymakers have started to recognize the seriousness of this issue. In 2002, in response to the case of Maggie McDonnell, a twenty-year-old college student who died after a driver who had been awake for thirty hours fell asleep, crossed three lanes of traffic, and crashed head-on into her car, New Jersey passed the first law criminalizing drowsy driving. Since this accident occurred before the law was instituted, the driver was fined $200 for careless driving.

Under the new law, a driver who gets into an accident after having been awake for more than twenty-four hours can be convicted of vehicular homicide. Since then, similar legislation has been proposed in at least four other states. The best advice is captured in a simple slogan: Drive alert, arrive alive.

CHAPTER 17

My Child Doesn't Sleep Well, So I Don't Either

Having a child gives you a new window into the world of sleep—from infancy through adolescence, you'll witness a steady progression of changes in your child's sleep habits. The good news is that from the fragmented sleep of the newborn, most children develop into good sleepers. They tend to fall asleep easily, sleep deeply through the night, and awaken feeling refreshed and energetic.

However, problems can arise if parents allow children to develop poor sleep habits. Most sleep issues in early childhood have to do with the establishment of routines and the interaction between child and parents. In this chapter, we'll look at what you can do to raise a healthy sleeper. Along with benefiting your child, this should make it easier for you to get sufficient sleep through these years as well (although during infancy, some parental sleep deprivation comes with the territory). Along the way, we'll look at some of the sleep-related issues that arise in each phase of childhood, such as sudden infant death syndrome (SIDS), difficulty getting your child to bed, nightmares and sleep terrors, early awakenings, and bed-wetting.

Newborns and Infants

Newborns sleep on and off around the clock, since their circadian rhythm of sleep and wakefulness has yet to develop fully. In between feedings, changings, and a lot of TLC, they sleep in chunks lasting from a few minutes to several hours, totaling as much as eighteen hours each day.

Although there's not much you can do to control when a newborn sleeps or doesn't, you can still start instilling good sleep habits. In Chapter 6 we talked about how positive associations with your sleep environment promote sleep, while negative associations can thwart it. These associations begin in infancy. A baby needs to learn that certain cues signal that it's time for sleep and that sleep occurs in certain places and not others.

The best way to start this is to put your baby to sleep when she's tired but not yet asleep. (For the sake of grammatical simplicity, I'm going to refer to the child as a female for this chapter, although the principles apply to both boys and girls.) This helps the child learn how to get to sleep by herself. If your baby gets used to falling asleep while being rocked or fed, she is likely to need that activity to fall back to sleep after waking up. So try to develop a routine that doesn't require you to be present for sleep to occur. It's OK to rock your baby to promote sleepiness—just try to stop before she actually falls asleep.

Bear in mind that it's normal for babies to wake up at night, since they get hungry every few hours. Breastfed babies generally wake up more often than formula-fed babies because breast milk is digested more quickly. To make nighttime wakings as brief as possible, comfort your child but don't play or do anything likely to stimulate her; if you do, you risk prolonging how long it takes her to get back to sleep. Often babies who wake at night to nurse will fall asleep quickly once their mothers are present. It's important to determine whether the baby is hungry or just requires nurturing for a few moments in order to fall back to sleep. The baby's mother can usually tell.

Cosleeping: Should We or Shouldn't We?

The practice of having a newborn share your bed at night is called *cosleeping* and has been the source of emotional debate for years. Advocates of cosleeping think it provides the newborn with a supportive emotional environment and promotes parent-child bonding, while others feel that sleeping in separate beds is safer, allows the baby to develop better and more independent sleep habits, and improves parent's sleep as well. The choice of whether or not to cosleep has been largely cultural, with cosleeping much less common in Western societies and more common in African communities.

How should you decide to choose? Cosleeping does not seem to have any psychological drawbacks but may have some physical ones. The American Academy of Pediatrics recommends against cosleeping to reduce the risk of SIDS. A 2006 study in the journal *Pediatrics* shows that sleep patterns develop differently depending on whether cosleeping is practiced. The authors compared three groups: one that practiced proximal care—essentially day-and-night, on-demand parental response with prolonged holding and cosleeping; one that followed schedules, routines, and separate sleeping; and one that was in between these two approaches. The different parenting approaches resulted in different child behavior. Children in the proximal care group had less fussing and crying during the day but had more nighttime waking and crying. Children who slept separately from their parents woke up less at night and disturbed their parent's sleep much less frequently. The rates of colic were the same in all groups, indicating that it is not a function of parenting but a physical disorder.

There are advantages and disadvantages to both approaches. I hope this information will help you decide whether cosleeping is the right choice for you.

Age Three Months to One Year

After a few months, nighttime feedings start to decrease, and by six months, many infants sleep through the night. From age three months to one year, infants typically sleep nine to twelve hours during the night and take up to four naps a day. The number of naps, which range from thirty minutes to two hours a day, decreases as the months go by. During this phase, parents have a more direct influence on how and when their babies sleep. There are a number of steps you can take to make sleep a positive experience.

As much as possible, keep your baby on the same daily schedule. Having the same times for waking, eating, napping, and playing will make her feel secure and comfortable and help make bedtime go smoothly. Also, it's vital to continue the practice of putting the baby to sleep when she is drowsy but not yet asleep. Babies who become accustomed to parental assistance at bedtime are more likely to cry for their parents to help them return to sleep during the night.

As the child becomes more aware of her surroundings, you can put more effort into making bedtime a special time. Go through a certain routine, such as having a light snack, bathing, cuddling, saying good night, and reading a story or singing a lullaby. At the end of the routine, the lights go off and it's time to fall asleep. Keep it short and simple—if you make too big a production of it, your baby may try to extend the routine. Baths can be playtime for young children and are often stimulating, not soothing. If this happens with your child, move the bath to the morning or more than two hours from the baby's desired bedtime. Also, make sure the routine can be used anywhere, so you can help her get to sleep when you visit friends and relatives.

It's also important to put some thought into finding your baby's ideal bedtime. In the evening, identify the hour when the child starts to slow down and get physically tired. Then make sure the bedtime routine is finished and she's in bed by that time, not afterward.

Remember that this is about your child's routine, not yours. Parents, especially in families where both parents work, may be tempted to keep their child up late so they have more time together. While well intentioned, this approach sets a pattern that can last into the school years and lead to sleep deprivation.

Some babies are soothed by the sound of a vaporizer or a fan running, since the white noise blocks out the distraction of other sounds. You can use ordinary appliances or purchase specially made white noise machines.

Sudden Infant Death Syndrome

During the first year of life, babies are at risk of sudden infant death syndrome, which is the leading cause of infant deaths. The peak risk time is between two and four months.

Although the cause of SIDS is unknown, it's likely due to the immaturity of infants' neurological system, which makes it difficult to react to situations in which breathing is hampered. Experts theorize that when babies' breathing is impaired, such as when their face is buried in the mattress, under covers, or in the sheets, they can't lift their head to improve breathing. Research has shown that preventing babies from sleeping on their stomachs significantly cuts the risk, so it's critical that you always put your baby to sleep on her back.

Colic

Although not actually a sleep disorder, colic is a common problem of infancy that can disturb sleep. The child is inconsolably fussy and screams (seemingly) endlessly in the late afternoon and evening. These episodes can interfere with daytime naps and make it difficult to get her to sleep at night.

Colic usually wanes by four months of age, but it can affect sleep habits for much longer if parents' attempts to soothe the child inadvertently interfere with the establishment of a regular sleep routine. If your child is colicky, first check with your physician to make sure no other medical problems explain the fussiness.

213

Reducing the SIDS Risk

In 1992, after evaluating a large number of studies conducted in Europe and Australia, the American Academy of Pediatrics (AAP) recommended keeping infants off their stomachs as a means to prevent SIDS (see Figure 17.1). This advice led to a dramatic reduction in the percentage of infant deaths caused by SIDS each year. In 2005, the AAP amended its policy to also recommend against putting babies to sleep on their side, based on research findings that they can roll onto their stomachs from the side position.

In addition, the AAP discourages parents from sharing their bed with the baby during sleep, due to the danger of an adult rolling onto the baby. Infants may be brought into the parents' bed for nursing or comforting but should be returned to their own crib or bassinet when the parents are ready to return to sleep.

The AAP also recommends allowing babies to use pacifiers at nap time and bedtime throughout the first year of life, based on research showing that pacifier use reduces the risk of SIDS. If you breastfeed your baby, wait until she is one month old to begin pacifier use to ensure that breastfeeding is firmly established. If the baby refuses the pacifier, do not force it on her, and do not reinsert it once she falls asleep.

Other AAP recommendations for reducing the SIDS risk include using a firm sleep surface, keeping soft objects and loose bedding out of the crib, and avoiding overheating the baby with too many

As long as colic's the cause, work to reestablish a normal sleep/wake routine as described earlier.

Trouble Falling or Staying Asleep

What to do when your baby won't go to sleep without crying or wakes up crying during the night is one of the most frequently discussed aspects of parenting. In most cases, this problem—known as childhood behavioral insomnia—is due to inappropri-

FIGURE 17.1 Optimal Sleeping Position for Infants

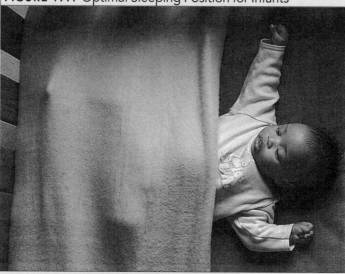

To reduce the risk of sudden infant death syndrome, babies should be put to sleep on their backs. If you use a blanket, it should reach no higher than the baby's chest, and you should tuck the ends under the crib mattress to ensure safety. Courtesy of the National Institutes of Health

layers of covers or a hot bedroom. To prevent flattening of the back of the head, place the infant on her stomach frequently when she's awake.

ate sleep associations or inadequate limit setting. It typically surfaces at about age six months, when you expect your baby to start sleeping through the night.

Sleep onset problems are typically due to the child developing reliance on unsuitable associations to fall asleep, such as rocking, the parents' bed, or the sound of a television. If the associated objects or conditions aren't present, the child cries. When parents restore the unsuitable conditions by allowing the child to sleep in their bed, driving the child around in the car, leaving the TV on, and so forth, they only prolong the problem.

The other common sleep onset problem is stalling and refusing to go to sleep. This often develops when parents fail to set effective limits, allow the child to delay bedtime, and don't establish a sleep routine.

The same problems can occur with nighttime awakenings. When children wake up during the night, they typically go right back to sleep. If the conditions associated with going to sleep are not present (such as the parent or rocking), then the child may be unable to fall back to sleep and will cry.

In the 1980s, Harvard Medical School's Dr. Richard Ferber developed an effective way to deal with these problems. His idea is an extension of the practice of putting a baby to sleep when sleepy but not yet asleep, which reestablishes a proper sleep routine and switches the sleep associations to more appropriate conditions for sleep.

You start by putting your child to sleep in bed and leaving the bedroom. If she cries, wait at least five minutes before you check on her. When you go back into the room, soothe the child with your voice but don't pick up, rock, or feed her. Gradually increase the amount of time that passes between checks. After a few days, the baby learns that crying earns nothing more than a brief check and learns to fall asleep on her own.

Dr. Ferber recommends using his method starting at age six months. Before you attempt it, make sure there are no external problems (illness, pain, medications, or the like) causing or contributing to your baby's crying.

Some parents find it difficult to stay outside the room while their baby cries. If this is the case, you may want to try a modified approach in which you stay in the room, sitting in a chair until she falls asleep. Using the same time increments, gradually move the chair farther and farther away from the bed until you're out of the room.

Rhythmic Movement Disorders

It's common for infants to try to soothe themselves with rhythmic movements such as body rocking, head rolling, or in extreme cases, head banging. The movements occur as the child is getting ready to drift off to sleep. Although the sound of the child's bed moving can be disturbing, in most cases, there are no negative health effects and medical intervention isn't necessary. The movements usually go away by age five. If you're concerned about injury or bothered by the sound, modify the baby's sleep environment, such as putting the child's mattress on the floor.

Toddlers

From ages one to three, toddlers need about twelve to fourteen hours of sleep every twenty-four hours. The number of naps continues to decrease and usually drops to one a day by eighteen months. During this phase, as toddlers grow more independent and increase their motor, cognitive, and social skills, it becomes more common for them to resist going to bed. Many experience separation anxiety. Some try to delay bedtime or refuse to go to bed altogether. They may express fears of monsters and climb out of the crib or bed.

You can minimize problems by continuing the good habits you've already established, such as maintaining a daily sleep schedule and a consistent bedtime routine. Never use sending your child to bed as a threat. Bedtime needs to be a secure, loving time, not a punishment. Your goal is to teach your child that bedtime is enjoyable, just as it is for us adults.

As language plays more of a role in your relationship, it becomes more important to set limits that are consistent, clearly communicated, and enforced. All parents want to comfort their children and protect them, but allowing them to change the bedtime routine by letting them stay up late or by sleeping in the child's bed will prolong, not solve, the problem.

During this time, toys become a key part of the child's life. To help with separation anxiety, you may also want to encourage the use of a security object such as a blanket, a doll, or a stuffed animal. However, don't go overboard and fill up your child's bed with toys, since too many objects in bed can be distracting and can create a choking hazard.

Early Awakenings

A common problem during this phase is that some toddlers consistently wake up an hour or two before you do and want your attention. This can happen for a number of reasons, so you need to be a bit of a detective to identify the cause. First, look for environmental factors that affect sleep. Check the bedroom for too much early-morning light or noise, and correct any problems you find. If the child always wakes up hungry, make sure she gets plenty to eat during the daytime, and try gradually delaying breakfast by ten minutes a day to break the association of waking and eating.

If light, noise, or hunger isn't the problem, take a closer look at sleep patterns. Excessive daytime napping may be the culprit. Try shortening the first (or morning) nap—just don't go past the point where your child gets overly fatigued during the daytime. Your child may be a short sleeper, requiring less sleep than other children. If so, it may help to delay bedtime. Again, do this ten minutes at a time, until bedtime is an hour later. If the child becomes sleepy during the day or naps lengthen, you've gone too far.

Finally, look at your child's expectations. Have you taught her to think wake-up time is the time to play with Mom and Dad? Instead, encourage her to entertain herself quietly until it's time to get up. As long as she's not in serious distress, don't rush immediately to her room at the first sound of activity. Gradually lengthen the time before you go in. Make sure she has toys to play with when she wakes. Let your child know what you expect by talking at bedtime about what she should do in the morning.

Be patient and don't expect perfection—few children are totally silent in the morning. Many sing or talk to themselves or make other noises. Keep in mind that there will be times when your child really needs you in the morning (in cases of sickness or injury, for example), so don't hesitate to go into her room in such instances.

Sleepwalking

This parasomnia (see Chapter 14) can occur anytime after the child begins to walk. Although scary to observe, sleepwalking is only of concern if the child seems at risk of harm. Just make sure the environment is as safe as possible. Children usually grow out of it; medication may be helpful in rare cases.

Preschoolers

Between the ages of three and five, children typically sleep eleven to thirteen hours each night. Some still nap and some don't. As with toddlers, difficulty falling asleep and waking up during the night are common, so you want to avoid introducing new factors that will disrupt sleep. For example, don't give your child drinks with caffeine in them, like tea or cola, and go easy on chocolate. Avoid the temptation to put a television in your child's bedroom. Research shows that watching TV at bedtime is linked to bedtime resistance and delays in falling asleep, especially if the set is in the child's room.

During this period, children want to be more independent, which can include trying to control bedtime. Continue to maintain a reasonable bedtime and a regular nighttime routine, promote proper sleep associations, and set effective limits on delaying behavior.

Nightmares and Sleep Terrors

This is the phase when nightmares and sleep terrors often become an issue. It's important for parents to be able to distinguish between the two and handle them in a way that disrupts sleep as little as possible.

Nightmares. Almost all kids have nightmares. They usually occur later in the night, during REM sleep, and they can be remembered at the time and in the morning. To prevent nightmares, discuss comforting things before bedtime and don't let your child watch violent or scary shows on television, especially right before sleeping.

When nightmares do occur, remain calm and reassuring, encourage your child to talk about it, and stay in the room until she settles down and is ready to go back to sleep. Don't get into bed with your child or allow her to get into yours—this sends the message that she should be afraid of her own bed, and it can turn into a habit that's difficult to break.

If nightmares happen more frequently or your child becomes afraid of going to sleep, then you need to address the issue during the day. Talk about what's frightening her and reassure her that the nightmares aren't real. But make sure to maintain a regular sleep routine and prevent bad habits from developing.

Occasionally, nightmares reflect more significant emotional problems. If this seems to be the case, talk to your pediatrician.

Sleep Terrors. About 3 percent of young kids experience sleep terrors—severe attacks of fear or panic during sleep that prompt them to sit up in bed and scream. Sleep terrors last only a few minutes, and the child rapidly returns to normal sleep. In the morning, she does not remember the episode.

It's easy to tell the difference between nightmares and sleep terrors: Nightmares don't prompt screams, they usually wake the child up, and they usually occur during the last few hours of sleep. Sleep terrors do trigger screams, don't wake up the child, and usually occur during the first few hours of sleep (often at the same time each night) during non-REM sleep.

If your child has sleep terrors, don't disturb or try to comfort her—since she's still actually asleep, this isn't beneficial. Instead, stay nearby and make sure she doesn't hurt herself. Being overtired and staying up too late can trigger sleep terrors, so you may

Case History

Jeremy was a bright and happy child who made friends easily and did well at school. So it was hard to understand why nighttime seemed so terrifying. Starting at a young age, he would frequently bolt upright in bed an hour after he went to sleep and let out a bloodcurdling scream.

At first, his parents and siblings would run to his side to see what was happening. Jeremy would have a terrified look on his face, but after a few minutes, he would lie down and go back to sleep. His family's efforts to calm him made no difference, and in the morning he never remembered a thing. This became such a common event that his brother and sister would just call out, "Everything's fine, Jeremy," and wait for him to go back to sleep.

Concerned that something was seriously wrong, Jeremy's parents came to see me. I reassured them that there was nothing wrong with their son and that things would get better as he grew up. Over time, the night terrors diminished, occurring only a few times a year. The only real problem was when friends would sleep over. If Jeremy's parents forgot to warn his friends, they would be terrified by the boy's screams—much more than Jeremy was. Eventually, the episodes ceased altogether.

be able to prevent them by making sure your child is getting enough sleep.

Although sleep terrors can be frightening, they aren't dangerous and typically aren't a sign of emotional distress. Children usually outgrow them after a few months or years. Be patient, and remember to warn babysitters and other family members who may be present overnight so they'll understand what's happening and won't overreact.

If nightmares or sleep terrors become so frequent that they prevent restful sleep, or if your child appears likely to harm herself, talk to your doctor.

Young Children

From ages six to twelve, children typically need ten or eleven hours of sleep. Most don't nap. Even though your child becomes more self-sufficient with each birthday, it's important to continue emphasizing the need for sleep, since this is the age when many kids start a trend toward becoming more and more sleep deprived, due to increasing demands on their time from school, sports, and other extracurricular and social activities. Through these years, you should periodically assess how much sleep your child needs. A child is getting the right amount if she can fall asleep within fifteen to thirty minutes, can wake up easily when it's time to get up, is awake and alert all day, and doesn't need a nap during the day.

If your child complains that her bedtime is earlier than her friends', explain that every child is different and that you're keeping her bedtime at the right time for her because it's healthy. Always remember that letting kids stay up late isn't doing them any favor.

Bed-Wetting

Bed-wetting, also called sleep enuresis, is extremely common among preschoolers. It's considered a problem, however, if it's still occurring by age six. Bed-wetting kids often experience psychological turmoil as a result of teasing from playmates and punishment or humiliation by ill-informed parents.

Statistically, 80 to 85 percent of children are consistently dry throughout the night by age five. After that, the number of children who continue to wet the bed decreases by about 15 percent per year, even without treatment, and only 1 to 2 percent of children still wet the bed by the time they're fifteen. Bed-wetting is more common in boys than girls.

There are two types of bed-wetting: primary and secondary. In primary, the child has never been consistently dry at night and wets the bed three or more times per week. In secondary, a child who has been dry at night for at least three to six months begins to occasionally wet the bed again.

Advanced Treatments for Bed-Wetting

When basic measures don't put an end to bed-wetting, more advanced techniques often will. There are several options:

- **Bed-wetting alarm.** You can purchase a device that includes an alarm attached to a sensor that is placed in the child's underwear. If the sensor gets wet, the alarm goes off, waking the child so he or she can get up and finish urinating in the bathroom. After several weeks or months of use, many kids learn to recognize when they need to urinate and achieve dryness.
- **Bladder training exercises.** Some bed wetters respond to bladder-retention training in which they're encouraged to hold their urine for longer and longer periods during the daytime to train the muscles of the bladder.
- **Medications.** As a last resort, medications can be used to treat bed-wetting, usually in conjunction with other therapies. One of the most common is desmopressin acetate (Concentraid, DDAVP, Stimate), a synthetic drug that is similar to the body's natural ADH. If the drug is successful in keeping the child dry for several months, it's tapered and eventually stopped. Some children use this medication to stay dry only when needed, such as when they're away at summer camp or at a friend's sleepover party.

  Anticholinergic medications such as oxybutynin (Ditropan) and tolterodine (Detrol), which relax bladder contractions and increase bladder volume, are also sometimes used. The antidepressant imipramine (Tofranil) was once used commonly but is rarely prescribed today.

Primary bed-wetting, also known as persistent bed-wetting, is the most common type, accounting for nine out of ten cases. It's believed to occur mostly for physiological reasons—bed wetters may not yet be able to recognize that their bladder is full, or they may not have developed enough control over the muscle that controls the bladder opening to stop urinating during sleep. In some children, areas of the brain that control arousal also may be affected, allowing them to sleep through a full bladder rather than waking up to urinate.

Hormones can also play a role. Under normal circumstances, the body's level of antidiuretic hormone (ADH), which decreases the production of urine by the kidneys, rises during sleep and causes the bladder to fill more slowly. In some children who wet the bed, this nighttime rise in ADH does not happen as expected. The amount of urine made remains the same as during waking hours, so the bladder continues to fill as much as it would during the daytime.

Primary bed-wetting seems to have a genetic basis, since having parents who were bed wetters as children significantly increases a child's chances of having the same problem. In 1995, researchers identified a particular chromosome as the home of the bed-wetting gene in some families.

Secondary bed-wetting can result from a variety of physical and psychological problems. A large percentage of children with secondary bed-wetting are under some type of emotional stress. Almost any change in the environment—good or bad—can be a trigger; for example, a new baby, a death in the family, parental divorce or marriage problems, or a new home or school. In other cases, bed-wetting is due to a medical problem, such as a urinary tract infection, diabetes, or a sleep arousal disorder such as sleep apnea. In these cases, there are usually other obvious symptoms of medical illness, and bed-wetting stops once the ailment is treated.

If your child is a chronic bed wetter, try these steps first:

- Provide encouragement and praise for dry nights—never punish, shame, or blame the child. Avoid embarrassing responses such as the use of diapers; diapers treat the bed, not the child.
- Remind your child to urinate before going to bed; if the child doesn't feel the need to go, tell her to try anyway.
- Limit liquids in the last two hours before bedtime, as well as foods that melt into liquids, such as ice cream and gelatin.

- Set up a "token and reward system" to motivate your child to stop wetting the bed. This typically involves using a colorful chart to keep track of progress, with a gold star for every dry night. When the chart is filled, give your child a new toy or a treat.

Keep in mind that even with progress, occasional accidents happen. It's vital that you remain calm as you change your child's sheets and underpants. Don't show disgust or disappointment. To make cleanup easier, place a rubber liner or large plastic bag under cloth sheets.

If bed-wetting continues, consult your pediatrician and consider more advanced treatment options.

Parasomnias

Parasomnias such as sleepwalking, sleep terrors, and nightmares tend to diminish during this time period. If they persist, increase, or lead the child into dangerous situations, see your physician or a sleep specialist.

Restless Legs Syndrome

RLS (see Chapter 12) is often misdiagnosed as "growing pains" when it begins during early childhood. It tends to run in families and can be related to problems with iron and dopamine metabolism. Treatment in children is similar to the treatment in adults.

Adolescents

Teens continue to need a lot of sleep (nine or ten hours), but it becomes increasingly hard for them to obtain it. This is due to the hectic pace of their lives (homework, jobs, sports, and so on) and the fact that their days must often start early even though their sleep/wake rhythm is oriented toward staying up late and sleeping late. Many maintain a constant sleep debt, leading them to nod off during classes.

Teens tend to be fiercely independent, but you can still play a role in encouraging healthy sleep habits. For starters, you can be a role model by making sleep a high priority for yourself. Next, now that your child is old enough to understand the scientific basis of sleep's role in health, you might try discussing the basics of sleep physiology, emphasizing that getting enough sleep will help socially and academically. Make sure your teen is aware of the risk of falling asleep at the wheel.

You can also create a sleep-friendly room for your teen that is cool, quiet, and dark. Discourage the use of the telephone and computer close to bedtime, and limit consumption of caffeinated beverages.

Next, keep an eye out for signs of insufficient sleep. They include difficulty waking up in the morning, irritability late in the day, falling asleep during quiet times of the day, and sleeping for extra-long periods on the weekends. If your teenager isn't getting enough sleep, have a talk about better ways to balance school, work, and social demands. Often these are tough choices, so it's important to really listen and make well-considered recommendations.

Be on the lookout for depression, one sign of which is staying in bed or sleeping more than usual. Other signs include feeling persistently sad, anxious, or hopeless for several weeks or months; losing interest in formerly enjoyable activities; experiencing a lack of energy, weight changes, and appetite disturbances; exhibiting moodiness, irritability, and restlessness; feeling guilty, helpless, or worthless; having difficulty concentrating, remembering things, and making decisions; withdrawing from friends or family; losing self-confidence and self-esteem; doing poorly in school; and thinking about death and suicide.

Delayed Sleep Phase Disorder

Many adolescents like to stay up late and sleep in late. While this results partly from a desire to engage in late-night social activities, the natural delay in the circadian sleep/wake rhythm at this age is often a factor as well. In some cases, teens who are unable to get to sleep at a reasonable time or who constantly have trouble getting up for school have full-fledged delayed sleep phase disorder.

Treatments to shift the circadian rhythm so it is more in line with the required daily schedule can help (see Chapter 15).

Narcolepsy

Narcolepsy can occur in children as young as age five, but it most commonly occurs during adolescence. Children with narcolepsy (see Chapter 13) suffer from extreme sleepiness and may experience uncontrollable sleep attacks several times a day, leading them to nod off while eating, talking, or even playing. Additional signs of early onset narcolepsy include great difficulty getting up in the morning and a tendency to become confused or aggressive upon waking. Children can also demonstrate cataplexy, the sudden loss of muscle tone during wakefulness, and temporary paralysis or vivid dreaming on falling asleep or awakening. Cataplexy is often described as fainting in young children. Narcolepsy is often misdiagnosed as a learning disability or attention deficit disorder, delaying treatment for many years.

Obstructive Sleep Apnea

Sleep apnea (see Chapter 11) can occur at any age from infancy to adolescence, but it's most commonly detected in older children and adolescents. Older children with sleep apnea usually snore loudly, and their parents often describe their breathing as heavy with pauses and snorts. Fragmentation of sleep can lead to sleepwalking, sleep terrors, and bed-wetting, and children may complain of morning headaches.

Although some kids with sleep apnea are extremely sleepy during the day, many are not. Instead, they can be irritable, hyperactive, and aggressive. Other daytime symptoms include poor school performance, frequent upper airway infections, and a general failure to thrive.

Often, childhood sleep apnea is caused by enlarged tonsils or adenoids. However, allergies, weight problems, and other medical problems also may contribute to it.

CHAPTER 18

Diagnosis: What to Expect from a Sleep Doctor or Sleep Center

By now, you've learned a lot about sleep disorders and their symptoms. You may suspect that you have a particular disorder or just know that something is wrong that isn't helped by ordinary measures such as improving sleep hygiene. Either way, you may benefit from seeing a sleep doctor, who can determine whether you have a sleep disorder and ensure that you get proper treatment if you do. In this chapter, we'll look at how physicians diagnose sleep disorders and what it's like to stay overnight at a sleep center.

When Should I See a Doctor About My Sleep?

I recommend a sleep evaluation for anyone who has the following problems:

- Trouble getting to sleep or getting restful sleep for more than a month or two
- Not feeling rested despite getting as much or more sleep than the amount that used to make you feel rested

- Falling asleep at inappropriate times during the day despite getting seven and a half to eight hours of sleep a night (This is particularly true for anyone who gets sleepy while driving.)
- Being told you snore loudly and gasp or stop breathing at night
- Having to sleep in a different room because your sleep is so disruptive to your bed partner
- Feeling there's still a problem after following the six-step plan outlined in Chapter 6

Before you see a sleep doctor, you'll probably see or at least talk with your regular doctor first. Primary care physicians (PCPs) can help with certain sleep problems. For example, when someone is sleeping badly following a death in the family or some other stressful event, a PCP can prescribe a medication for short-term use.

Primary care doctors can also play an important role in weeding out other health problems that may be the true source of a person's sleep difficulty. Physicians may screen problem sleepers for symptoms of depression, anxiety, physical or sexual abuse, or other psychological problems or traumatic experiences. If one of these conditions is diagnosed, a PCP may make a referral to a psychologist or psychiatrist for treatment. Since they're already familiar with their patients' medical history, PCPs are in a good position to diagnose and treat physical problems such as diabetes and arthritis that may be disrupting sleep.

However, primary care doctors are not well trained about sleep medicine and have a mixed track record when it comes to recognizing sleep disorders that aren't caused by other health issues. Perhaps because sleep medicine is a relatively new discipline, most don't ask their patients much about sleep or recognize the signs of many sleep disorders. This is partly due to a lack of training in sleep matters and partly because they're busy seeing so many patients with a variety of health problems. As a result, many do not routinely consult with experts in sleep medicine.

A Brief History of Sleep Medicine

Although descriptions of sleep and sleep problems go back to the beginning of written history, the study of sleep did not really take off until the twentieth century. Nathaniel Kleitman, a physiology professor at the University of Chicago, ushered in the era of sleep discovery in the 1920s by studying the effects of sleep deprivation and describing the various internal events that occur during sleep.

The first sleep center, the narcolepsy clinic at Stanford University under the direction of Dr. William Dement, was established in 1964. Recognition of other disorders and the practice of sleep medicine began to grow in the 1970s, and the first specialty exam for sleep specialists was given in 1978. With an extensive body of scientific knowledge, more than eighty recognized sleep disorders, and more than twenty-six hundred sleep specialists in the United States, sleep medicine was recognized as an official medical subspecialty in 2005.

This means that if you suspect you have a sleep disorder, it's up to you to bring this up with your doctor and ask for a referral to a sleep specialist—something many people are hesitant to do. Even people with chronic sleep problems rarely bring up sleep during their medical visits. In my practice, people have often had sleep problems for many years before they finally come to my clinic.

In some areas, such as rural towns far from academic medical centers, it may be hard to find a sleep specialist. For a list of accredited sleep centers and the board-certified sleep specialists who work there, go to sleepeducation.com.

Seeing a Sleep Doctor

The sleep doctor's first task is to learn as much as he or she can about your usual sleep habits and your current sleep problem.

Once you make an appointment, you'll be asked to fill out a detailed questionnaire in advance of your first meeting. The following sample questionnaire shows you the kinds of questions that are typically included. It's often helpful to have your bed partner help with some of the questions, since you may not know all the things you do while you're asleep.

Sample Sleep History Questionnaire

Describe your sleep problem.

How long have you had trouble sleeping, and what do you think started the problem? Did it come on suddenly?

What time do you go to bed, and when do you wake up?

How long does it take you to fall asleep?

Once you're asleep, do you sleep through the night or wake up frequently?

Do you wake up feeling rested?

How much sleep do you think you get each night?

Is your bedroom dark and quiet?

What do you do in the few hours before bedtime?

Do you follow the same sleep pattern during the week and on weekends? If not, how are weekends different?

How well do you sleep on the first few nights when you're away from home?

At home, do you sleep better in your bedroom or in another room in the house?

Do you often feel sleepy during the day?

Do you fall asleep at inappropriate times or places?

Have you ever been in a car accident or had a close call because you've nodded off at the wheel?

Do allergies or nasal congestion bother you at night?

Do you have physical aches and pains that interfere with sleep?

What medications or drugs (including alcohol and nicotine) do you use? Have you ever taken sleep medications? If so, which ones?

Do you ever feel discomfort or a fidgety sensation in your legs and feet when you lie down? Do you have to get up and walk around to relieve the feeling? Are the sensations worse in the evening?

Do you kick or thrash around at night?

Have you ever been told you stop breathing in your sleep or
awaken because it's hard to breathe?

Does your bed partner or roommate mention that you snore loudly
or gasp for air at night?

Do you ever awaken with a choking sensation, indigestion, or a
sour taste in your mouth?

Have you felt excessively worried, anxious, or depressed over the
last month?

Have you been treated for anxiety or depression?

You may also receive a sleep diary to fill out for a week before
your appointment. This is a way to graphically show much of the
same information from the questionnaire. You'll note your bedtime; how much sleep you got at night; how often you woke up
during the night; your morning wake-up time; whether you
napped in the daytime; and when you exercised, drank caffeinated
beverages and alcohol, and took medication.

When you meet with the sleep doctor, he or she will review
your questionnaire and sleep diary with you and ask follow-up
questions. To get an accurate picture of what factors may be
affecting your sleep, he or she is likely to ask about recent changes
in your residence, job, marital status, children, pets, and other
possible stress-related issues.

Next, the doctor may assess your sleepiness by seeing how you
rate on what's known as the Epworth sleepiness scale. This step is
crucial, since people are often bad at judging this phenomenon
themselves. Many people are so used to sleep deprivation that they
don't realize how tired they are; instead, they may see themselves
as lazy, lethargic, or unmotivated. Or they may not think it's
unusual to fall asleep at a movie or while sitting at dinner with
friends.

The test is simple. You imagine yourself in the eight situations
listed, selecting your likelihood of dozing in each one using this
scale: 0 = would never doze; 1 = slight chance of dozing; 2 =
moderate chance of dozing; 3 = high chance of dozing.

Home-Based Sleep Tests

Some sleep-monitoring equipment can be used at home. The information collected is less reliable for diagnosis and treatment, so an overnight stay at a sleep center is preferred. However, portable recordings can be useful if polysomnography is not available in a person's area, or if a patient is bedridden and cannot be moved. Home-based tests may also be used as a follow-up tool to an overnight stay when a physician wishes to evaluate a treatment's effectiveness. Two types of equipment are most commonly used.

- **Wrist actigraphy.** A wristwatch-sized monitoring device that automatically records arm or leg movements can be used to track periods of sleep and wakefulness over long periods of time (typically about a week). This can be helpful in evaluating circadian rhythm disorders. Although it cannot determine the stage of sleep, the device can help clarify ambiguous aspects of a sleep diary, such as entries reporting long hours of sleep but exhaustion during the day. The actigraphy device may reveal that brief awakenings during the night are unknowingly

_____ Sitting and reading

_____ Watching TV

_____ Sitting inactive in a public place, like a theater or a meeting

_____ As a passenger in a car for an hour without a break

_____ Lying down to rest in the afternoon

_____ Sitting and talking to someone

_____ Sitting quietly after lunch (when you've had no alcohol)

_____ In a car while stopped in traffic

Generally, a total of 10 points or higher is cause for concern. Also, the less appropriate the circumstances (such as when stopped in traffic while driving or during a conversation), the more dangerously sleepy you are considered to be.

disturbing sleep. In some studies, wrist actigraphy accurately determined the person's sleep/wake cycle almost 90 percent of the time.

- **Apnea detectors.** To detect breathing disturbances during sleep, a patient can be equipped with apnea detectors that can measure heart rate, snoring sounds, body position, nasal airflow, and the amount of oxygen in the blood. These devices can miss mild apnea and other sleep disruptions, and they don't provide the information about other aspects of sleep that's needed to rule out other sleep disturbances, so they should only be used when the patient's physician is familiar with the devices' benefits and limitations and has experience interpreting the results.

Less commonly, full polysomnography can be done in the home, with all the usual sleep study equipment packed into a small suitcase. A technologist may need to visit the home to set up the equipment before the patient goes to sleep. Full polysomnography can be helpful in evaluating a broader range of sleep disorders.

The sleep doctor will also ask you about your medical history, family history, and health habits (diet, exercise, smoking, and so on) and may perform a physical exam.

If you have any questions during your appointment, don't hesitate to ask. Sleep doctors are familiar with just about everything that can occur during sleep or as a result of it, so there's no reason to be bashful.

Based on all the information obtained, the sleep doctor will decide whether you need a sleep study. There's a good chance you won't—insomnia and circadian rhythm disorders, for example, can be diagnosed by a thorough history and physical examination alone.

During the initial evaluation, if I suspect a sleep disorder such as narcolepsy, periodic limb movement disorder, sleep apnea, or one of the parasomnias, I recommend formal sleep testing. A sleep study confirms the diagnosis and shows how severe the problem is. Determining the severity of any disease is important because it's one of the necessary factors in selecting the best treatment. In some cases, when something precludes the possibility of coming into the sleep center, I might suggest a patient use home-based equipment to assess his or her sleep.

The Sleep Center

There are more than 850 sleep disorders centers and laboratories accredited by the American Academy of Sleep Medicine. Accreditation means these centers have met rigorous standards and provide the highest quality of care. Most sleep doctors are affiliated with sleep centers or have one to which they commonly send patients for testing.

Staying overnight at a sleep center usually costs between $800 and $1,500. Most health insurance companies will cover most or all of the cost if you have a referral from a sleep doctor—check with your insurer to find out how your plan handles this.

Once you have an appointment, the center may send you a sleep diary to fill out in advance of your visit, if you haven't filled one out previously.

On the day of your sleep study, avoid caffeine and alcohol after 12 P.M. and try not to nap. It's OK to shower and wash your hair with shampoo, but do not apply hair sprays, oils, or gels—the slickness can interfere with the sleep-monitoring equipment.

You should pack an overnight bag, as you would for an overnight stay at a hotel or a friend's house. Bring your own nightclothes and a favorite pillow from home if you have one. You might also want to bring a book or a magazine to read during downtime (but don't go overboard and bring office work or handheld games). If you have any other special needs, advise the sleep center staff in advance so they can accommodate them. You can take your regular medications, but the staff will need to know what they are.

You're usually asked to arrive in the early evening, around seven or eight. If you're expecting the center to have an impersonal, institutional feel, you're in for a surprise—most are homey and comfortable, like a small hotel. A technologist will greet you and show you to your bedroom, which is nearly always a private room with a bathroom attached.

Once you're settled in, there may be some final paperwork for you to complete. You may also view a video or DVD that explains what will occur during the night.

Next, you'll change into your nightclothes. After you take some time to relax, a technician will start setting up the sleep-monitoring equipment. You should inform the technologist of any recent changes in your sleep or specific problems you've been having in the days leading up to the visit.

Recording Your Sleep

Sleep centers use what's known as polysomnography to make a continuous record of your sleep. About two dozen small, wafer-thin electrodes and other sensors are pasted on specific body sites to take a variety of readings during the night. They may be placed in the following locations:

- On your scalp to track brain waves
- Under your chin to measure fluctuations in muscle tension (called an electromyogram, or EMG)
- Near your eyes to measure eye movements
- Near your nostrils to measure airflow
- On your earlobe or finger to measure the amount of oxygen in your blood (using a device called an oximeter)
- On your chest to record heart rate and rhythm
- On your legs to record twitches or jerks
- Over your rib muscles or around your rib cage and abdomen to monitor breathing

Readings are collected on a single computer file (called a polysomnogram) that can be analyzed as they're recorded and later

FIGURE 18.1 Preparation for Sleep Study

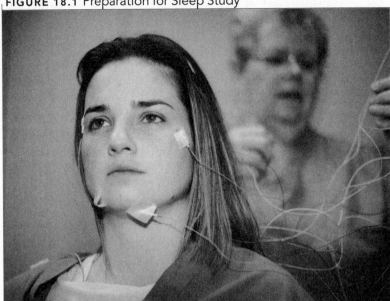

During a sleep study, a continuous record is made of the person's sleep. Information is gathered from about two dozen wafer-thin electrodes and other sensors pasted on specific body sites.   Copyright © Scientifica/Visuals Unlimited

on. Figure 18.1 shows a person being prepared for a sleep study. The procedure is not painful, and once you get accustomed to it, you'll notice the sensors and recording less than you might initially suspect. You will be able to roll over and change positions almost as easily as you would at home because the electrode wires are gathered in a kind of ponytail behind your head. Most people don't find all the equipment an obstacle to falling asleep.

In addition, audiotape equipment may be used to record snoring, talking during sleep, or other sounds. A videotape may also be recorded to compare with the polysomnogram. This may show, for example, that you snore only when in a certain position. Signs of movement disorders (such as periodic limb movement disorder) or parasomnias are usually apparent on the video.

Once all the equipment is set up, you'll be left alone to fall asleep. Throughout the night, laboratory staff will monitor the

FIGURE 18.2 Monitoring the Sleep Study

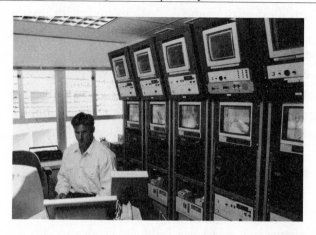

While a patient undergoes a sleep study, laboratory staff examine the readings from a nearby control room.

instruments in a nearby control room (see Figure 18.2). Bedrooms are equipped with automatic intercoms, so if you need to go the bathroom, all you need to do is say this out loud. All the wires attached to you are plugged into a box, so the technician will come in and unplug you from the box, freeing you to get up.

If a breathing problem is detected early on, you may be awakened and given continuous positive airway pressure during the second half of the night. This allows the sleep experts to monitor how well the treatment works for you.

In cases in which narcolepsy is suspected, the sleep doctor may also want to assess your daytime sleepiness. If so, you'll need to stay for most of the next day. In this case, you'll be told in advance, so you can make appropriate plans. You'll probably want to bring extra reading materials that will help you pass the time.

You'll take the multiple sleep latency test (MSLT), which measures how long it takes you to fall asleep while lying down in a quiet room and identifies what stages of sleep occur during a brief nap. The procedure is usually repeated four or five times during the day at two-hour intervals. Your sleep patterns will be monitored with most of the same recording equipment used the night before. Falling asleep within five minutes each time indicates extreme sleepiness.

An alternate way to measure daytime sleepiness is the maintenance of wakefulness test (MWT). Here, you're given the opposite instructions from an MSLT: try to stay awake. Your ability to do so is also affected by the degree of sleep deprivation or fragmentation you experience.

In most cases, the overnight stay is sufficient. You'll be awakened at about 7 A.M., and the technician will remove the monitoring equipment. Then you can shower and wash your hair to remove the paste used to attach the electrodes and head home.

Getting Your Diagnosis

You won't leave the sleep center the next morning with the final results from your study. First, technologists must score the huge amount of data generated during the study, and the sleep doctor must review and interpret the results, a labor-intensive process that can take a week to ten days. Then the sleep doctor discusses the results with you during a follow-up appointment or over the phone. There are three general possibilities:

- You may find out that you're actually sleeping better than you thought and don't need treatment. Some people who are convinced they get little or no sleep during the night are surprised to learn that they're getting six, seven, or even a full eight hours of sleep, a phenomenon known as paradoxical insomnia. This doesn't mean their stay was in vain—gaining this knowledge can ease anxiety and ultimately lead to better health. This discovery can also steer your doctor toward other explanations for your problem.
- You may receive a specific diagnosis of one of the sleep disorders—those most commonly diagnosed after a sleep

study are sleep apnea, PLMD, and narcolepsy. If so, the sleep doctor will review the relevant treatment options and make arrangements for you to begin therapy.

- In rare cases, the results are inconclusive and you may be asked to spend another night at the center.

I have seen thousands of patients in my career and am always amazed at the number who suffer sleep problems for years before seeking help. I hope this chapter has illustrated that sleep doctors and sleep centers will take your problem seriously, determine what is wrong, and offer treatments capable of improving your sleep.

CHAPTER 19

Health Conditions and Medications That Disrupt Sleep

To this point, we've focused mostly on problems with sleep and wakefulness that result from primary sleep disorders such as insomnia, sleep apnea, and narcolepsy. However, many sleep-related problems result from "nonsleep" illnesses—such as heart failure, diabetes, and Alzheimer's disease—or from medications used to treat these illnesses. In most cases, treating the underlying disorder is the key to improving sleep. In this chapter, we'll review the common health conditions and medications that can make it hard to sleep at night or stay awake during the day.

Cardiovascular Disease

Congestive heart failure and coronary artery disease are the two most common heart problems that affect sleep.

Congestive Heart Failure

Congestive heart failure is a condition in which the heart can no longer meet the body's need for blood because it's pumping inefficiently. This causes a backup of blood in the veins to the heart, leading the kidneys to retain fluid and the body's tissues to swell. The swelling, or edema, most commonly affects the legs, but it can also occur in the lungs and other tissues and organs.

When edema in the lungs occurs during the night, people may awaken feeling short of breath. Using pillows to elevate the upper body may ease this problem.

Heart failure patients also can be awakened just as they are falling asleep by a characteristic breathing pattern called Cheyne-Stokes respiration, a form of central sleep apnea in which a series of increasingly deep breaths is followed by a brief cessation of breathing. Treating the heart failure and improving the effectiveness of the heart is the best treatment. Some people may need to use supplementary oxygen, a positive airway pressure device, or a diuretic medicine called acetazolamide to help them breathe and sleep more normally. In mild cases, benzodiazepine sleep medications can help some people sleep through these episodes.

In addition, congestive heart failure raises an individual's risk for obstructive sleep apnea, which can disrupt sleep, cause daytime sleepiness, and worsen heart failure. Chapter 11 discusses sleep apnea treatments.

Coronary Artery Disease

Coronary artery disease is the buildup of fatty deposits and fibrous tissue inside the arteries that supply blood to the heart. This buildup, called atherosclerosis, can cause the coronary arteries to become significantly narrower, which decreases the blood supply to portions of the heart muscle and triggers a specific type of chest pain called angina.

Angina often occurs during the overnight hours, which disrupts sleep. It can generally be treated with medications such as nitrates, beta blockers, calcium channel blockers, and aspirin. If medication isn't effective, angioplasty or coronary artery bypass surgery may be necessary.

Complete blockage of the arteries causes a heart attack, the damage and death of heart muscle otherwise known as a myocardial infarction (MI). Circadian factors affect the timing of heart attacks, with the highest frequency occurring between 6 A.M. and noon. Obstructive sleep apnea changes the timing of them, with more heart attacks and death occurring between midnight and 6 A.M. in OSA patients.

Endocrine Disorders

Endocrine disorders that commonly affect sleep include diabetes and thyroid disease.

Diabetes

Diabetes is a common disorder that affects the way the body processes and uses carbohydrates, fats, and proteins. Each of these nutrients is a source of glucose (sugar), which is the most basic fuel for the body. The clearest sign of diabetes is a high level of sugar in the blood.

People with uncontrolled diabetes are often awakened by night sweats or a frequent need to urinate. Controlling blood sugar with a combination of exercise, dietary changes, and medication can reduce sleep problems. If diabetes has damaged nerves in the legs—a condition called neuropathy—nighttime movements or pain may also disturb sleep, and the likelihood of developing restless legs syndrome increases. Several types of medication are available to treat diabetic neuropathy.

Thyroid Disease

Thyroid hormones, which are produced by the thyroid gland in the lower front of the neck, regulate the body's energy level. When levels of thyroid hormones are unusually high, a condition known as hyperthyroidism, the body burns energy faster and many vital functions speed up.

Hyperthyroidism can make it hard to fall asleep, and night sweats cause nighttime arousals. The most common treatment is radioactive iodine, which stops excessive production of thyroid

Coping with Frequent Nighttime Urination

A frequent need to get up and go to the bathroom at night is called nocturia. Nocturia is a common cause of sleep loss, especially among older adults, affecting nearly two-thirds of people between the ages of fifty-five and eighty-four at least a few nights per week.

A mild case causes a person to wake up at least twice during the night; in severe cases, a person may get up as many as five or six times. Not surprisingly, this can lead to significant sleep deprivation and daytime fatigue.

Nocturia becomes more common with age. As we get older, our bodies produce less of the antidiuretic hormone that enables us to retain fluid. With decreased concentrations of this hormone, we produce more urine at night. Also, the bladder tends to lose holding capacity as we age, and older people are more likely to suffer from medical problems that affect the bladder.

Nocturia has numerous possible causes, including some of the disorders covered in this chapter (such as heart failure and

hormones. The medications propylthiouracil, methimazole (Tapazole, Thiamazole), and beta blockers also are used to treat hyperthyroidism.

In other instances, levels of thyroid hormones can be abnormally low, a condition known as hypothyroidism. Feeling cold and sleepy during the daytime is a hallmark of this disorder. People with low thyroid levels tend to gain weight and their muscles don't work as well as they should; both situations can bring about obstructive sleep apnea. Hypothyroidism can be treated with replacement doses of synthetic thyroid hormones.

Because thyroid function affects every organ and system in the body, the symptoms can be wide-ranging and sometimes difficult to decipher. If you suspect you have a thyroid disorder, ask your doctor for a blood test.

diabetes), other medical conditions (such as urinary tract infection, enlarged prostate, liver failure, multiple sclerosis, and sleep apnea), and medication (especially diuretics). Some cases are caused or exacerbated by excessive fluid intake after dinner, especially drinks containing alcohol or caffeine.

Treatments for nocturia fall into one of three categories: correction of medical causes, behavioral interventions, and medication. The first step is to try to identify the cause and correct it. If your physician can find no medical reason for the condition, try behavioral approaches such as cutting down on how much you drink in the two hours before bedtime, especially caffeine and alcohol. If the nocturia persists, your doctor may prescribe one of a growing number of medications approved to treat an overactive bladder. The most commonly used is desmopressin, which mimics some of the action of the antidiuretic hormone. If your problem is increased or you experience more frequent contractions of the bladder, relaxant agents such as tolterodine (Detrol) and oxybutynin (Ditropan) can be effective.

Neurological Disorders

Parkinson's disease, epilepsy, Alzheimer's disease, and headaches are among the neurological disorders that may affect sleep.

Parkinson's Disease

Parkinson's disease is a central nervous system disorder that causes problems with body motions, including tremors, muscle stiffness, slowed body movements, unstable posture, and difficulty walking. It occurs when neurons in a part of the brain called the substantia nigra gradually die. These cells normally produce dopamine, a chemical that helps relay messages between areas of the brain that control body movement. Abnormally low levels of dopamine make it difficult for a person with Parkinson's disease to control muscle tension and movement. REM sleep behavior disorder (see

Chapter 14) can be an early sign of nervous system degeneration and often precedes the other symptoms of Parkinson's.

People with this disease frequently have difficulty getting enough sleep. Just getting in and out of bed can be a struggle. A bedrail or an overhead bar (known as a trapeze) can help with mobility problems.

Sleep itself is disrupted by the disease. Parkinson's patients frequently have sleep onset insomnia and, once asleep, wake up frequently. Some arousals are from the tremors and movements, but others seem to result from the disorder itself. As a result, daytime sleepiness is common. Sometimes these problems can be treated with medication, but the dosage must be strictly monitored because some drugs can worsen Parkinson's symptoms.

Levodopa, the mainstay of Parkinson's treatment, causes some patients to develop severe nightmares. However, the use of levodopa at night is important to maintain the mobility needed to change positions in bed.

Epilepsy

Epilepsy is a condition that causes recurrent, sudden, brief changes in the normal electrical activity of the brain. During an epileptic episode, commonly called a seizure or convulsion, brain cells fire uncontrollably at up to four times their normal rate, temporarily affecting the way a person behaves, moves, or thinks.

People with epilepsy are twice as likely as others to suffer from insomnia, and about one in four people with epilepsy have seizures that occur mainly at night, causing disturbed sleep and daytime sleepiness. Nocturnal seizures are often mistaken for sleep parasomnias or psychiatric disorders because of the outward similarities (such as bizarre behavior and vocalizations). Antiseizure drugs can cause sleepiness and changes in sleep architecture at first but tend to correct the sleep disturbances when used over time.

Sleep deprivation can also trigger a seizure, a phenomenon noted in college infirmaries during exam periods. Each semester, a few students suffer their first seizures after staying up late to study.

Alzheimer's Disease/Dementia

Alzheimer's disease is a disorder that impairs the brain's intellectual functions (memory, orientation, and calculation). Memory gradually deteriorates, causing impaired judgment and other problems that affect a person's ability to perform normal daily activities. Alzheimer's disease is the most common cause of dementia, accounting for more than half of all cases in people age sixty-five and older.

Alzheimer's disease and other forms of dementia may disrupt sleep regulation and other brain functions. Sleep is usually fragmented, with more awakenings and more time spent awake as the night progresses. Deep sleep is reduced, and REM sleep is less well organized. Wandering, disorientation, and agitation during the evening and night, a phenomenon known as sundowning, can require constant supervision and place great stress on caregivers. In such cases, benzodiazepine drugs or small doses of antipsychotic medications such as haloperidol (Haldol) and thioridazine (Mellaril) are often helpful. However, these drugs should be used carefully since they can also increase disorientation and falls.

Headaches

Two types of headaches—migraines and cluster headaches—may be related to changes in the size of blood vessels leading to the brain cortex. Pain occurs when the walls of the blood vessels dilate. People who are prone to headaches should try to avoid sleep deprivation, as lack of sleep can promote headaches. Researchers theorize that as the body catches up on missed sleep, it spends more time in deep sleep (when vessels are most constricted), making the transition to REM sleep more dramatic and likely to induce a headache. Pain relievers and other medications can be used to treat these headaches.

Strokes/Tumors

Sleepiness coupled with dizziness, weakness, headache, or vision problems may signal a serious problem such as a brain tumor or stroke, which requires immediate medical attention. In addition, strokes and obstructive sleep apnea are closely intertwined. Having OSA increases your risk for developing a stroke, and rates of OSA are much higher immediately following a stroke.

Respiratory Disease

Breathing problems such as asthma and chronic obstructive pulmonary disease may cause sleep difficulties.

Asthma

Asthma is a chronic lung condition that causes breathing difficulties and wheezing when air passages become inflamed and narrow. Some people have only occasional, mild symptoms, while others have nearly constant symptoms with severe, life-threatening flare-ups.

Circadian-related changes constrict the airway during the overnight hours, often causing nocturnal asthma attacks that rouse the sleeper abruptly. Breathing difficulties or fear of having an attack may make it more difficult to fall asleep. One study found that nearly 75 percent of people with asthma experienced frequent awakenings every week. Medications (bronchodilators and anti-inflammatory drugs) can usually control asthma attacks, reducing nighttime awakenings. However, they have stimulant side effects and may cause difficulty falling asleep.

Chronic Obstructive Pulmonary Disease

COPD refers to a group of disorders that damage the lungs and make breathing increasingly more difficult over time. The two most common forms of COPD are chronic bronchitis and emphysema. In more than 80 percent of cases, the illness is related to cigarette smoking.

People who have emphysema or chronic bronchitis may find it difficult to fall and stay asleep because of excess sputum production, shortness of breath, and coughing. These symptoms can be eased with medications such as bronchodilators and cortico-steroids, allowing better sleep.

Those with severe disease are prone to drops in blood oxygen (hypoxemia) when the respiratory rate and breath size drop during sleep, especially during REM sleep. The low oxygen levels can cause sleep fragmentation and promote heart disease. Hypoxemia is treated with supplemental oxygen therapy.

Mental Illness

Mental health problems such as anxiety, depression, and schizophrenia often lead to poor sleep.

Anxiety

Severe anxiety, formally known as generalized anxiety disorder, is a mental illness that causes a person to have persistent, nagging feelings of worry, apprehension, or uneasiness. These feelings are unusually intense and out of proportion to the person's actual troubles.

People with generalized anxiety disorder tend to be hyperalert and frequently have trouble falling and staying asleep, and they often do not feel rested when they awake. A combination of psychotherapy and antianxiety medication (including benzodiazepines and antidepressants) can ease anxiety, leading to better sleep.

Depression

Depression is a mood disorder with symptoms such as extreme sadness, a sense of despair, irritability, a lack of pleasure or interest in pleasurable activities, and a loss of energy. Almost 90 percent of people with serious depression wake up earlier than desired, and some have difficulty falling asleep or wake up frequently during the night. In chronic low-grade depression, insomnia or sleepiness may be the most prominent symptom. Lab studies have shown that people who are depressed spend less time in deep sleep and may enter REM sleep more quickly at the beginning of the night.

Depression can be treated with a combination of psychotherapy and medication, and successful treatment often improves sleep.

Bipolar Disorder

Bipolar disorder, which used to be called manic depression, is a mental disorder characterized by severe mood swings. During a manic episode, an individual may not sleep at all for several days. This is often followed by a "crash" during which the person spends most of the next few days in bed. Bipolar disorder is treated with a combination of psychotherapy and medication (the mood-stabilizing drug lithium, anticonvulsants, antidepressants, and antipsychotics), which usually helps patients sleep.

Schizophrenia

Schizophrenia is a chronic mental illness in which people may have difficulty recognizing reality, thinking logically, and behaving normally in social situations. Some people with schizophrenia sleep very little when they enter an acute phase of their illness. Their sleep patterns are likely to improve between episodes. Even so, many schizophrenics rarely obtain a normal amount of deep sleep. Schizophrenia is usually treated with antipsychotic medication, and antianxiety drugs and antidepressants may be used as well. A treatment's effect on sleep varies widely by patient.

Seasonal Affective Disorder (SAD)

SAD is a phenomenon in which the reduced amount of sunlight in the wintertime leads to depression. Researchers speculate that people with SAD produce too much melatonin (or are extrasensitive to normal amounts of this drowsiness-inducing hormone) and don't make enough serotonin.

People with SAD sleep more than normal, struggle to get out of bed, and may still feel sleepy and lethargic during the day. Bright light therapy in the morning (see Chapter 15) may alleviate SAD symptoms. Antidepressants also can be helpful.

Other Health Problems

A number of other health problems can also negatively affect sleep.

Gastroesophageal Reflux Disease (GERD)

GERD is a digestive disorder in which the stomach's juices (acid and digestive enzymes) flow backward, or reflux, into the esophagus. The lining of the esophagus is not equipped to handle these caustic substances, so it becomes inflamed, causing heartburn and other symptoms.

Lying down in bed often worsens heartburn and disrupts sleep. You may be able to avoid this problem by abstaining from heavy or fatty foods, as well as coffee and alcohol, in the evening. You can also use gravity to your advantage by elevating your upper body with the use of an under-mattress wedge or by placing blocks under the bedposts. Just using extra pillows is not enough. Over-the-counter and prescription drugs that suppress stomach acid secretion can also help.

Kidney Disease

In kidney disease, the kidneys lose their ability to filter enough waste products from the blood and to regulate the body's balance of salt and water. Eventually, the kidneys slow their production of urine or stop producing it completely.

Kidney disease can cause waste products to build up in the blood and insomnia or RLS often occur. Severe cases of kidney disease are treated with dialysis or a transplant, but this does not always return sleep to normal. When sleep problems persist, medication for insomnia or RLS may be needed.

Arthritis

Arthritis pain can make it hard for people to fall asleep and to resettle when they shift positions. In addition, treatment with corticosteroids frequently causes insomnia. Taking aspirin or a nonsteroidal anti-inflammatory drug (NSAID) just before bedtime to relieve pain and joint swelling may help a patient sleep.

Medications That Disturb Sleep and Wakefulness

In many cases, medication rather than illness is the culprit behind sleep problems. A number of drugs are common sleep robbers, while others may cause unwanted daytime drowsiness.

As we review these medications, bear in mind that side effects do not occur in all people and that their severity varies considerably by individual. In some cases, side effects are an unavoidable cost for receiving the benefit the drug provides. In others, your doctor may be able to suggest alternatives that do not affect sleep or to reduce the dosage so there's less sleep disruption.

Cardiovascular Drugs

Drugs to control hypertension and other heart problems are among the most commonly prescribed. Many of them affect sleep and daytime alertness.

- **Alpha blockers.** These hypertension medications, which act on nerve cells that respond to the neurotransmitter norepinephrine, can cause daytime drowsiness and fatigue as well as insomnia and nightmares. Alpha blockers include clonidine (Catapres) and methyldopa (Aldomet).
- **Antiarrhythmics**. These drugs, used to treat heart rhythm problems, cause daytime fatigue in up to 10 percent of patients. Antiarrhythmics include disopyramide (Norpace) and diltiazem (Cardizem).
- **Beta blockers.** Beta blockers are used to treat high blood pressure, arrhythmias, and angina. Up to 4 percent of patients find that these drugs make it hard to fall or stay asleep or cause nightmares. Commonly used beta blockers include atenolol (Tenormin), metoprolol (Lopressor), and propranolol (Inderal).

- **Diuretics.** Diuretics, which rid the body of excess sodium and water, are used to treat hypertension, heart failure, and other disorders. They can interfere with sleep by inducing urination throughout the night. In addition, potassium deficiency, a common side effect of some diuretics, can cause painful nocturnal cramping of calf muscles.

Antidepressants

Antidepressants are now frequently prescribed to treat insomnia, and many people find that they help. However, a small but significant percentage of people who take antidepressants for emotional problems find the drugs actually worsen insomnia. The class of antidepressants known as selective serotonin reuptake inhibitors is most often problematic, with 10 to 20 percent of patients reporting insomnia. SSRIs include fluoxetine (Prozac), sertraline (Zoloft), paroxetine (Paxil), citalopram (Celexa), fluvoxamine (Luvox), and escitalopram (Lexapro). Other classes of antidepressants, such as tricyclics and monoamine oxidase inhibitors, also may cause insomnia.

Tricyclics and SSRIs can bring on or worsen RLS and periodic limb movements, leading to daytime sleepiness. In addition, certain antidepressants—including the serotonin modulators nefazodone (Serzone) and trazodone (Desyrel) and the tetracyclic mirtazapine (Remeron)—are associated with increased daytime drowsiness. If you take antidepressants, be sure to report any side effects you experience to your doctor so he or she can work with you to find an effective regimen.

Other Drugs

Other medications that commonly affect sleep include the following:

- **Beta agonists.** Beta agonists are used to treat COPD and asthma attacks. They can cause insomnia; the most commonly prescribed is albuterol (Ventolin, Proventil).

- **Corticosteroids.** Corticosteroids such as prednisone relieve inflammation. In addition to being used for respiratory disorders such as asthma and allergies, they're prescribed to treat injuries, arthritis, intestinal disorders, and many other ailments. They frequently cause insomnia and daytime jitteriness.
- **Nicotine patches.** Patches used to curb smokers' cravings deliver small doses of nicotine into the bloodstream around the clock. People who use them often suffer insomnia or experience disturbing dreams.
- **Sedating antihistamines.** Over-the-counter antihistamines such as Benadryl, commonly taken to relieve cold or allergy symptoms, cause drowsiness in most people. If you're taking a sedating antihistamine and are bothered by drowsiness, your physician may recommend a nonsedating alternative that does not readily enter the brain and affect wakefulness and sleep.
- **Stimulants.** Sympathomimetic stimulants—such as dextroamphetamine (Dexedrine), methamphetamine (Desoxyn), methylphenidate (Ritalin), and pemoline (Cylert)—are powerful central nervous system stimulants that enhance the effect of brain chemicals involved in wakefulness. They're used to treat attention deficit disorder, narcolepsy, and other disorders. People taking these agents may experience insomnia, and once asleep, they get less deep sleep. When the drug is discontinued, extreme sleepiness and REM sleep rebound may follow.
- **Theophylline.** Theophylline, used to treat asthma, bronchitis, and emphysema, can cause insomnia.
- **Thyroid replacement drugs.** Synthetic forms of hormones are used to treat hypothyroidism. These drugs, including levothyroxine (Synthroid, Levoxyl), liothyronine (Cytomel), and liotrix (Thyrolar), may cause insomnia at higher doses.

Good Night and Good Luck

I hope this book has given you a better understanding of the critical role sleep plays in overall health. If you have trouble sleeping, I encourage you to seek help. It's important not to give up and to remember that help is available. Whatever the cause of your sleep difficulty, effective treatment exists that can work for you. Whether it's behavioral therapy, CPAP, medication, or something else, I can't tell you how many times patients who have struggled for years ultimately experience major improvement when their problem is correctly diagnosed and treated. Better sleep means better health. Sleep well.

Additional Resources

Organization	Provides Information On	Website
Aetna InteliHealth	General health and disease topics, including sleep	intelihealth.com
American Academy of Sleep Medicine	Sleep education, general sleep information, sleep centers	sleepeducation.com
American Insomnia Association	Insomnia	americaninsomniaassociation.org
American Sleep Apnea Association	Sleep apnea	sleepapnea.org
Harvard Health Publications	Newletters; special reports; books on general health and disease topics, including sleep	health.harvard.edu
Narcolepsy Network	Narcolepsy	narcolepsynetwork.org
National Center on Sleep Disorders Research	Sleep disorders and related research	www.nhlbi.nih.gov/about/ncsdr
National Sleep Foundation	Sleep medicine and related research, sleep centers	sleepfoundation.org
PubMed Central	Scientific research, including abstracts of published studies on sleep	pubmedcentral.nih.gov
Restless Legs Syndrome Foundation	Restless legs syndrome and periodic limb movement disorder	rls.org
U.S. Food and Drug Administration	Health-related news, including drug and device safety related to sleep	www.fda.gov
U.S. National Library of Medicine	Scientific research, including abstracts of published studies on sleep	www.nlm.nih.gov

Index

Acupuncture, 120–21
Adolescents
    delayed sleep phase disorder
        and, 226–27
    encouraging healthy sleep
        habits for, 225–26
    narcolepsy and, 227
    sleep and, 41–42
    sleep apnea and, 227
Adulthood
    sleep and, 42–45
    sleep changes during, 43
Advanced sleep phase disorder
        (ASP), 73, 74, 181. *See also*
        Delayed sleep phase disorder
        (DSP); Sleep disorders
    symptoms of, 182–85
    treatments for, 185–89
Aging, sleep and, 43, 45–48, 49
Alcohol use, 50, 58, 63–64
    obstructive sleep apnea and,
        126
Alertness, sleep and, 37–38
Alpha blockers, 254
Alpha sleep, 13–14
Alprazolam (Xanax), 102
Alternative insomnia treatments,
        115–16. *See also*
        Medications, sleep
    acupuncture, 120–21
    herbal supplements, 116–19
    hot baths, 121
    synthetic melatonin, 119–20

Alzheimer's disease, 78, 249
Ambien (zolpidem), 105–7, 112,
        178
    sleep eating and, 106
Animals, sleep needs of, 30
Antiarrhythmics, 254
Anticonvulsants, for RLS, 149,
        150–51
Antidepressants, 255
    for insomnia, 107–9
    for narcolepsy, 162, 163
    for obstructive sleep apnea,
        138
Antihistamines, 100–101
Anxiety
    medications for, 102–3
    sleep and, 251
Apnea. *See* Sleep apnea
Apnea detectors, 235
Architecture, sleep, 18–19
Arendt, Josephine, 195
Arthritis, 74, 253–54
Asthma, 250
Ativan (lorazepam), 102
Automatic behavior, 33
Awakenings, 72–73
    early-morning, 73–74
    toddlers and, 218–19

Babies. *See* Infants; Newborns;
    Toddlers
Barbiturates, 110
Baths, hot, 121

Bed-wetting
  advanced treatments for, 223
  primary, 222–24
  secondary, 222, 224
  young children and, 222–25
Bedrooms, 60
  creating optimal environments
    for, 61–62
Behavioral treatments, for
    insomnia, 83–93
  cognitive therapy, 92–93
  reconditioning, 85–87
  relaxation techniques, 88–91
  sleep hygiene, 85
  sleep restriction, 87–88
Benzodiazepine hypnotics,
  102–5
Benzodiazepine receptor
    agonists, 101–7
  benzodiazepine hypnotics,
    102–5
  nonbenzodiazepine hypnotics,
    105–7
Benzodiazepines, for RLS, 149,
  150
Beta agonists, 255
Beta blockers, 254
Bi-level PAP, 137
Bimodal circadian rhythms, 20
Biofeedback, 91
Bipolar disorder, 252
Bladder training exercises, 223
Bootzin, Richard, 85
Brain waves
  alpha pattern of, 13–14
  patterns of, 12
  patterns of, during sleep, 14
  recording, 12
  size and frequency of, 12
  sleep and, 11–13
Breathing disorders. See Sleep
  apnea; Snoring
Bright light therapy, 186–89
Bruxism, 78, 178–79

Caffeine, 62–63, 203
Cardiovascular diseases, that
  affect sleep, 243–45
Cataplexy, 156–57
Central sleep apnea (CSA),
  140–41. See also Obstructive
  sleep apnea (OSA); Sleep
  apnea
Chamomile, 118–19
Childhood, sleep and, 39–42
Childhood behavioral insomnia,
  214–16
Children, young
  bed-wetting and, 222–25
  parasomnias and, 225
  RLS and, 225
  sleep and, 41
  sleepwalking and, 169
Chronic insomnia, 81–82
Chronic obstructive pulmonary
  disease (COPD), 74,
  250–51, 255
Chronic pain, 72
Chronic secondary insomnia, 83
Chronotherapy, 186
Circadian rhythms, 20, 24
  bimodal, 20
  of body temperatures, 31
  free-running, 183
  homeostatic drives and, 24–26
Clonazepam (Klonopin), 102, 174
Cluster headaches, 249
Cognitive behavioral therapy
  (CBT), 93
Cognitive therapy, 92–93
Colic, 213–14
Comorbid insomnia, 83
Complete sleep deprivation,
  32–34
Confusional arousals, 77, 171–72
Congestion, snoring and, 124
Congestive heart failure, 243–44
Continuity of sleep, measuring,
  44

Continuous positive airway pressure (CPAP), 125, 136–37
Coronary artery disease, 244–45
Corticosteroids, 256
Cosleeping, 211
Cramps, sleep-related leg, 144
Creativity, sleep and, 38
Cumulative sleep debt, 24

Dalmane (flurazepam), 102, 104
Daytime drowsiness, 28–29, 74–75
Deacon, Stephen, 195
Death rates, amount of sleep and, 5
Deep breathing, 89–90
Deep sleep, 15–16
Deep sleep parasomnias, 168–72. See also Parasomnias
  confusional arousals, 171–72
  sleep terrors, 170–71
  sleepwalking, 168–70
Delayed sleep phase disorder (DSP), 71, 76, 120, 181. See also Advanced sleep phase disorder (ASP); Sleep disorders
  adolescents and, 226–27
  case history of, 184–85
  symptoms of, 182–85
  treatments for, 185–89
Dement, William, 231
Dementia, 249
Dental devices
  for obstructive sleep apnea, 137
  for snoring, 127–29
Dependence, sleep medications and, 98–99, 100–101
Depression, 73, 76, 251
Diabetes, 245
Diaphragmatic breathing, 89–90
Diaries, sleep, 233

Diazepam (Valium), 102
Diet, 57–58
Disorders. See Sleep disorders
Diuretics, 255
Doctors, primary care, 230. See also Sleep doctors
Dopamine agents, for RLS, 148–59
Doral (quazepam), 102, 104
Dreaming sleep. See Rapid eye movement (REM) sleep (dreaming sleep)
Dreams
  importance of, 16–17
  remembering, 50–51
Driving
  drowsy, 7, 204–7
  sleep deprivation and, 6
Drowsiness, daytime, 28–29, 74–75

Early-morning awakenings, 73–74
Eating disorders, sleep-related, 177–78
Education, sleep, 7
Effectiveness, sleep medication and, 96–97
Electroencephalogram (EEG), 12
Electromyogram (EMG), 237
Emphysema, 72
Endocrine disorders, that affect sleep, 245–46
Epilepsy, 78, 248
Epworth sleepiness scale, 233–34
Estazolam (ProSom), 102
Eszopiclone (Lunesta), 105, 107
Excessive daytime sleepiness (EDS), 74–75, 156
Exercise, 56–57

Ferber, Richard, 216
Flip-switch theory, of sleep, 154, 155

Fluid intake, 64
Flurazepam (Dalmane), 102, 104
Fluvoxamine (Luvox), 109
Free-running circadian rhythms, 183
Freud, Sigmund, 16

Gamma-aminobutryric acid (GABA), 101
Garcia, Jerry, 131
Gastroesophageal reflux disease (GERD), 72, 253
Grogginess, 99

Habits, maintaining good sleep, 58–61
Halcion (triazolam), 102
Hallucinations, hypnagogic, 157
Headaches, 249
Health
  lack of sleep and, 5–6
  sleep and, 35–36, 38, 54
Heart failure, 73, 76
Heartburn, 64–65
Herbal treatments, 116–19
  chamomile, 118–19
  lavender, 118
  passionflower, 119
  valerian, 117–18
Hi-tech treatments, for sleep disorders, 8
Home-based sleep tests, 234
Homeostasis
  circadian drives and, 24–26
  sleep and, 23–24
Hormone replacement therapy (HRT), 96–97
Hot baths, 121
Humans, sleep needs of, 30
Hygiene, sleep, 85
  for jet lag, 194
Hyperarousal, 72
Hyperthyroidism, 72, 245–46
Hypnagogic hallucinations, 157

Hypocretin, 154
Hypothyroidism, 75, 246

Infants. See also Newborns; Toddlers
  optimal sleeping position for, 215
  SIDS and, 213, 214
  sleep and, 40, 212–13
Insomnia, 70–72. See also Sleep disorders
  behavioral treatments for, 83–93
  case histories of, 86–87, 102–3
  childhood behavioral, 214–16
  chronic, 81
  classifications of, 81–83
  defined, 79–81
  FDA-approved benzodiazepine medications for, 102
  paradoxical, 71–72
  primary, 82
  rebound, 98
  secondary, 83
  short-term, 81
  as sleep disorder, 4
  sleep maintenance, 72, 73
  Sunday, 80–81
  transient, 81
  treatments for. See Alternative insomnia treatments; Medications, sleep
Insomniacs, 51–52
Internal clock, 19–20
  location of, 21
  zeitgebers for, 22

Jet lag
  factors for, 192–93
  minimizing, 193–96
  severity of, 191–93

Kidney disease, 73, 76, 253
Kleitman, Nathaniel, 231
Klonopin (clonazepam), 102, 174

L–tryptophan, 116–17
Larks, sleeping pattern, 31
Laser-assisted uvulopalatoplasty
    (LAUP), 128–29
Lavender, 118
Learning, sleep and, 52
Leg cramps, sleep-related, 144
Lifestyles, adopting healthy,
    56–58
Light, as cue for internal clock,
    22
Light boxes, 188
Light therapy, 186–89
Liquids, intake of, 64
Long sleepers, 29–30
Lorazepam (Ativan), 102
Lunesta (eszopiclone), 105, 107
Luvox (fluvoxamine), 109

Maintenance of wakefulness test
    (MWT), 240
Mandibular advancing devices,
    127–28
Mechanical dilators, 127
Medications, for bed-wetting,
    223
Medications, for movement
    disorders, 148–51
Medications, for narcolepsy,
    161–64
Medications, sleep, 8, 95–96. See
    also Alternative insomnia
    treatments
  amount spent on, 5
  author's perspective on
    prescribing, 110–13
  dependence and, 98–99,
    100–101
  effectiveness and, 96–97
  impact on sleep quality and,
    97–98
  for jet lag, 195
  over-the-counter, 99–101
  prescription, 101–10

rebound insomnia and, 98
  safety and, 99
  side effects and, 99
  tolerance and, 98, 100–101
  for treating ASP and DSP, 189
Medicine, sleep
  brief history of, 231
  training in, 7
Meditation, 90
Melatonin
  as cue for internal clock,
    22–23
  synthetic, 119–20, 195–96
  for treating ASP and DSP, 189
Melatonin receptor agonists, 109
Memory, sleep and, 38
Menopause, sleep and, 96–97
Microsleeps, 33
Migraines, 249
Modafinil (Provigil), 138, 163
Morning hangover, 99, 100
Movement disorders. See
    Periodic limb movement
    disorder (PLMD); Restless
    legs syndrome (RLS)
Movement disorders, rhythmic,
    217
Multiple sleep latency test
    (MSLT), 239–40
Muscle tone, snoring and, 124
Myths, about sleep, 49–54

Naps/napping, 53, 60
  shift work and, 202
Narcolepsy, 74. See also Sleep
    disorders
  adolescents and, 227
  case history of, 158–59
  causes of, 153–55
  diagnosing, 159–61
  living with, 164–65
  medical treatments for, 8
  medications for, 161–64
  symptoms of, 155–59

Nasal steroid sprays, for snoring, 127
Nasal strips, 127
Neurological disorders, that affect sleep, 247–50
Neuromuscular diseases, 75
Newborns. *See also* Infants
  cosleeping with, 211
  sleep and, 39–40, 210
Nicotine patches, 256
Nicotine use, 64
Nightmares, 77, 175–76
  case history of, 221
  medications that increase frequency of, 176
  preschoolers and, 220
Nocturia, 246–47
Nocturnal eating syndrome, 177–78
Non-REM sleep (quiet sleep), 13–16. *See also* Rapid eye movement (REM) sleep (dreaming sleep); Sleep
  alpha sleep and, 13–14
  Stage 1 of, 14
  Stage 2 of, 15
  Stage 3 of, 15–16
  Stage 4 of, 15–16
Non-twenty-four-hour sleep-wake syndrome, 183
Nonbenzodiazepine hypnotics, 105–7

Obesity, snoring and, 124
Obstructive sleep apnea (OSA), 123, 130–31. *See also* Central sleep apnea (CSA); Sleep apnea
  adolescents and, 227
  causes of, 131–33
  medications for, 137–38
  noninvasive treatment of, 135–38
  screening for, 134
  surgical treatments for, 138–40
  symptoms and signs of, 133–35
Older persons, sleep and, 45–46
Opiates, for RLS, 149, 150
Orexin, 154
Over-the-counter sleep medications, 99–101
Overactivation, 70, 72
Overnight sleep centers. *See* Sleep centers
Owls, sleeping pattern, 31

Palatal implants, 129, 139
Paradoxical insomnia, 71–72
Paralysis, sleep, 157
Parasomnias, 76–78, 106. *See also* specific parasomnia
  deep sleep, 168–72
  REM, 172–76
  young children and, 225
Parkinson's disease, 78, 247–48
Partial sleep deprivation, 34–35
Partners, sleeping with people who have sleeping disorders, 4–5, 78
Passionflower, 119
Patterns
  alpha, 13–14
  brain wave, during sleep, 14
Performance, sleep and, 37–38
Periodic limb movement disorder (PLMD), 73, 75
  about, 151–52
  medications for, 149
  treating, 152
Physicians, primary care, 230. *See also* Sleep doctors
Pills, sleeping. *See* Medications, sleep
Polysomnography, 234–35, 237–38
Positive airway pressures (PAP), 8, 135–37
Pregnancy, sleep and, 46–47

Preschoolers
  sleep and, 40–41
  sleep disorders of, 219–21
Prescription sleep medications,
    101–10. *See also* Alternative
    insomnia treatments;
    Insomnia; Medications, sleep
  antidepressants, 107–9
  barbiturates, 110
  benzodiazepine receptor
    agonists, 101–7
  melatonin receptor agonists,
    109
Presleep routines, 59–60
Primary bed-wetting, 222–24
Primary care doctors, 230. *See
    also* Sleep doctors
Primary insomnia, 82
Progressive muscle relaxation,
    89
ProSom (estazolam), 102
Provigil (modafinil), 138, 163

Quality of life, sleep deprivation
    and, 6
Quazepam (Doral), 102, 104
Questionnaires, sleep history,
    232–33
Quiet sleep. *See* Non-REM sleep
    (quiet sleep)

Ramelteon (Rozerem), 109
Rapid eye movement (REM)
    sleep (dreaming sleep),
    17–18. *See also* Sleep
  newborns and, 40
RBD. *See* REM sleep behavior
    disorder (RBD)
Rebound insomnia, sleep
    medications and, 98
Reconditioning, 85–87, 88
Relaxation techniques, 88–91
  biofeedback, 91
  deep breathing, 89–90

  meditation, 90
  progressive muscle relaxation,
    89
  visualization, 90–91
REM parasomnias
  nightmares, 175–76
  REM sleep behavior disorder
    (RBD), 172–75
REM sleep. *See* Rapid eye
    movement (REM) sleep
    (dreaming sleep)
REM sleep behavior disorder
    (RBD), 77, 172–75
  case history of, 174–75
Reproductive cycles, sleep and,
    46–47
Respiratory diseases, that affect
    sleep, 250–51
Restless legs syndrome (RLS)
  about, 143–47
  insomnia and, 71
  medications for, 8
  as sleep disorder, 4
  treating, 148–51
  young children and, 225
Restoril (temazepam), 102
Rhythmic movement disorders,
    217
RLS. *See* Restless legs syndrome
    (RLS)
Routines, presleep, 59–60
Rozerem (ramelteon), 109

Safety, sleep medications and, 99
Saper, Clifford, 154
Schizophrenia, 251
Seasonal affective disorder
    (SAD), 252
Secondary bed-wetting, 222,
    224
Secondary insomnia, 83
Sedating antihistamines, 256
Selective serotonin reuptake
    inhibitors (SSRIs), 255

Shift work, 71, 72–73, 75
  about, 196–200
  case history of, 199–200
  coping strategies for, 200–204
  at sleep labs, 199
Short sleepers, 29
Short-term insomnia, 81
Side effects, sleep medications
    and, 99
SIDS. See Sudden Infant Death
    Syndrome (SIDS)
Six-step plan, for sleep, 55–65
Sleep, 3–4. See also Non-REM
    sleep (quiet sleep); Rapid eye
    movement (REM) sleep
    (dreaming sleep)
  adolescents and, 41–42
  in adulthood, 42–45
  aging and, 43, 45–48
  architecture, 18–19
  average hours Americans, 5
  benefits of, 37–38
  brain waves and, 11–13
  cardiovascular diseases that
      affect, 243–45
  in childhood, 39–42
  circadian rhythms and, 20,
      24–26
  deep, 15–16
  dreaming. See Rapid eye
      movement (REM) sleep
      (dreaming sleep)
  endocrine disorders that affect,
      245–46
  flip-switch theory of, 154, 155
  health and, 54
  healthy lifestyles and, 35–36
  history, questionnaires for,
      232–33
  homeostatic drive for, 23–26
  lack of, and health problems,
      5–6
  learning and, 52
  medications that disturb,
      254–56

  menopause and, 96–97
  mental health problems that
      affect, 251–52
  myths about, 49–54
  neurological disorders that
      affect, 247–50
  older persons and, 45–46
  quiet. See Non-REM sleep
      (quiet sleep)
  recording, 237–40
  reproductive cycles and, 46–47
  respiratory diseases that affect,
      250–51
  six-step plan for, 55–65
  slow-wave, 15–16
  types of, 13
Sleep apnea, 73, 74–75, 76, 78.
      See also Central sleep apnea
      (CSA); Obstructive sleep
      apnea (OSA); Sleep disorders
  case history of, 125
  as disorder, 4
  equipment for monitoring,
      235
  positive airway pressure for, 8,
      135–37
  surgery for, 8
Sleep centers, 8, 236–40
  getting diagnosis from,
      240–41
  shift work at, 199
Sleep continuity, measuring, 44
Sleep debt. See also Sleep
      deprivation
  cumulative, 24
  repaying, 36–37
Sleep deprivation, 6. See also
      Sleep debt
  complete, 32–34
  cost of, 6
  driving and, 6
  health and, 34–35
  partial, 34–35
  quality of life and, 6
  role of, in catastrophes, 6

Sleep diaries, 233
Sleep disorders. *See also* specific
 sleep disorder
 cost of, 5–6
 diagnosing, 7–8
 hi-tech treatments for, 8
 as increasing problem, 5
 partners of people with, 4–5
 setting realistic expectations
  for solving, 8–9
 statistics on, 4–5
 treatment of, 6–7
Sleep doctors
 seeing, 231–36
 when to see, 229–31
Sleep drives, 25
Sleep eating, 106
Sleep eating disorders, 177–78
Sleep education, 7
Sleep enuresis. *See* Bed-wetting
Sleep evaluations, 229–30
Sleep fragmentation, 72
Sleep habits, maintaining good,
 58–61
Sleep hygiene, 85
 for jet lag, 194
Sleep inertia, 75–76
Sleep maintenance insomnia, 72,
 73
Sleep medications. *See*
 Medications, sleep
Sleep medicine
 brief history of, 231
 training in, 7
Sleep-monitoring equipment,
 234
Sleep needs, 27–29
 calculating one's, 28–29
 of humans vs. animals, 30
Sleep paralysis, 157
Sleep quality, sleep medications
 and, 97–98
Sleep-related eating disorders,
 77
Sleep-related leg cramps, 144

Sleep restriction, 87–88
Sleep terrors, 77, 170–71
 case history of, 221
 preschoolers and, 220–21
Sleep tests, home-based, 234
Sleep timing, disturbances of. *See*
 Advanced sleep phase
 disorder (ASP); Delayed
 sleep phase disorder (DSP)
Sleep/wake rhythms, 19–20
Sleepers
 larks, 31
 long, 29–30
 owls, 31
 short, 29
 standard, 30–31
Sleeping pills. *See* Medications,
 sleep
Sleepwalking, 77, 168–70
 toddlers and, 219
Slow-wave sleep, 15–16
Smoking, 64
Snoring, 50, 78, 123
 causes of, 124–26
 nonsurgical treatments for,
  126–28
 oral appliances for, 8
 prevalence of, 124
 as sleep disorder, 4
 surgery for, 128–30
Somnambulism, 77, 168–70, 219
Somniloquy, 177
Somnoplasty, 129, 139
Sonata (zaleplon), 105–7, 112
SSRIs (selective serotonin
 reuptake inhibitors), 255
Stage 1, of non-REM sleep, 14
Stage 2, of non-REM sleep, 15
Stage 3, of non-REM sleep,
 15–16
Stage 4, of non-REM sleep,
 15–16
Stimulant medications
 for narcolepsy, 161–63, 162
 sleep and, 256

Stimulus control, 85–87
Strokes, 249–50
Sudden Infant Death Syndrome
    (SIDS), 213, 214
  optimal sleeping position for
      reducing risk of, 215
Sunday insomnia, 80–81
Suprachiasmatic nucleus (SCN),
    21–22, 109
Synthetic melatonin, 119–20
  for jet lag, 195–96

Talking in one's sleep, 177
Teenagers. *See* Adolescents
Teeth grinding. *See* Bruxism
Temazepam (Restoril), 102
Terrors, sleep, 77, 170–71
  case history of, 221
  children and, 219–21
Theophylline, 256
Thyroid disease, 245–46
Thyroid replacement drugs, 256
Time cues, for internal clock, 22
Timing, sleep, disturbances of.
    See Advanced sleep phase
    disorder (ASP); Delayed
    sleep phase disorder (DSP)
Tobacco use, 64
Toddlers
  naps and, 217
  sleep and, 40
  sleep problems of, 217–19
Tolerance, sleep medications and,
    98, 100–101
Total sleep deprivation, 32–34
Tracheostomy, 139–40
Transient insomnia, 81

Treatments, hi-tech, for sleep
    disorders, 8
Treatments, insomnia. *See*
    Alternative insomnia
    treatments
Triazolam (Halcion), 102
Tumors, 249–50
Two-peaked pattern circadian
    rhythm, 20

Uvulopalatopharyngoplasty
    (UPPP), 128
  for OSA, 139

Valerian, 117–18
Valium (diazepam), 102
Visualization, 90–91

Wake after sleep onset (WASO),
    44
White, Reggie, 131
Wrist actigraphy, 234–35

Xanax (alprazolam), 102
Xyrem (sodium oxybate), 163–64

Young children
  bed-wetting and, 222–25
  parasomnias and, 225
  RLS and, 225
  sleep and, 41
  sleepwalking and, 169

Zaleplon (Sonata), 105–7, 112
Zeitgebers, 22–23, 183
Zolpidem (Ambien), 105–7, 112,
    178

About the Authors

Lawrence J. Epstein, M.D., attended medical school at George Washington University in Washington, D.C., followed by an internal medicine residency and chief residency at the VA Medical Center in West Los Angeles. He then completed a pulmonary, critical care, and sleep medicine fellowship at Cedars-Sinai Medical Center in Los Angeles. Dr. Epstein is board certified in sleep medicine, internal medicine, pulmonary diseases, and critical care medicine. He has been practicing sleep medicine since 1992, having served as the military consultant on sleep disorders to the Air Force surgeon general and as the medical director of the Sleep Medicine Laboratory at the West Roxbury VA Medical Center. He is currently regional medical director for Sleep HealthCenters, a sleep medicine specialty practice group with multiple sites in Boston. He is on the faculty at Harvard Medical School as an instructor in medicine with dual appointments in the division of sleep medicine and the pulmonary division at Brigham and Women's Hospital. He was the president of the American Academy of Sleep Medicine from 2005 to 2006.

Steven Mardon is a freelance writer specializing in health issues who has written for newsletters, newspapers, and magazines for more than ten years. A graduate of Boston University, he previously worked as a reporter at the *Poughkeepsie Journal* and as a medical writer for *Hippocrates*, a magazine for physicians, and *HealthNews*, a newsletter for consumers. He is coauthor of *The Harvard Medical School Guide to Healing Your Sinuses* with Ralph B. Metson, M.D.